CW00323141

Return to an Address of the
Honourable the House of Commons dated
22 July 2002 for the

Foot and Mouth Disease 2001:
Lessons to be Learned Inquiry Report

Chairman, Dr Iain Anderson CBE

Presented to the Prime Minister and the Secretary of State for Environment,
Food and Rural Affairs, and the devolved administrations in Scotland and Wales

Ordered by the House of Commons *to be printed*
22 July 2002

LONDON: The Stationery Office

HC 888   £10.00

CONTENTS

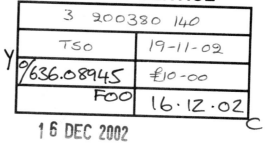
USE OF ABBREVIATIONS

Throughout this report we have tried not to use too many abbreviations and acronyms. Those we have used are as follows:

COBR   Cabinet Office Briefing Room

DEFRA   Department of the Environment, Food and Rural Affairs

FMD   Foot and Mouth Disease

MAFF   Ministry of Agriculture, Fisheries and Food

NFU   National Farmers' Union

OIE   Office International des Epizooties

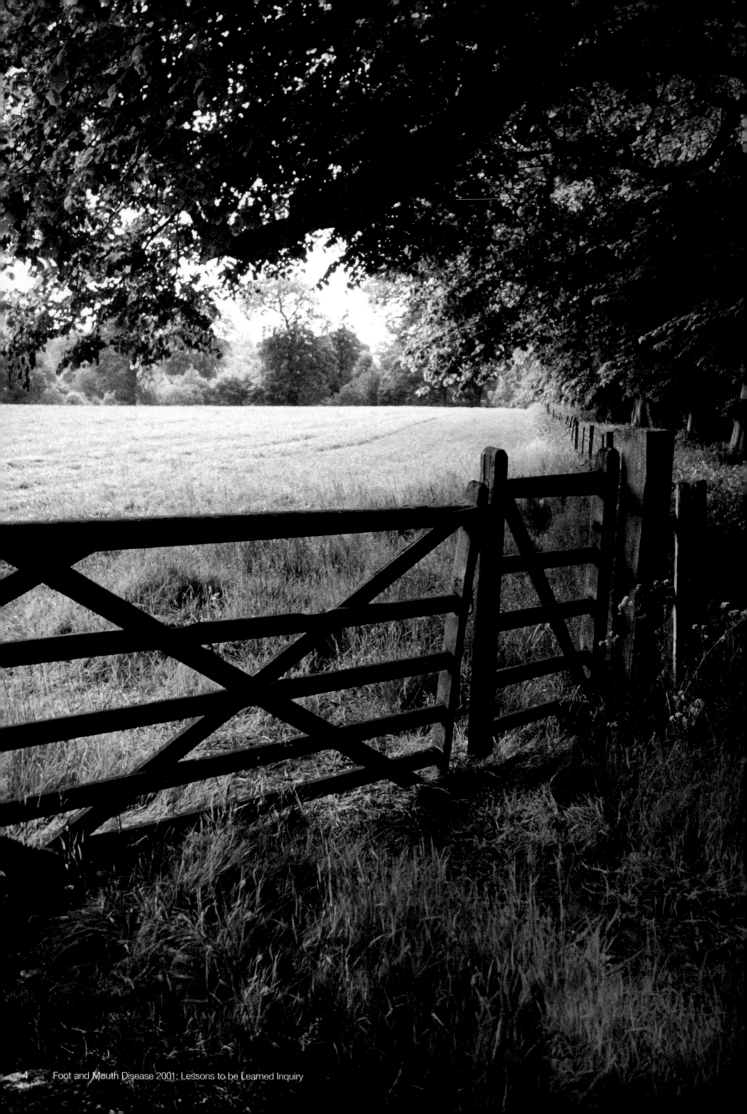

1 FOREWORD BY IAIN ANDERSON

In August 2001 I was asked by the Prime Minister and the Secretary of State for Environment, Food and Rural Affairs to conduct an Inquiry into the Government's handling of the outbreak of Foot and Mouth Disease (FMD) in Great Britain during 2001 in order to draw out lessons and make recommendations. I was asked to start when the epidemic was judged to be over and then to report within six months.

I appointed a small secretariat (Appendix 18.7) to organise the programme of work and assemble the facts. This team was led by Alun Evans, a senior civil servant with experience across government at the highest levels.

The Inquiry gathered its facts in a variety of ways. We asked for written submissions and received 576. We travelled around the country, visiting many of the worst hit regions. In the course of these visits we held public meetings, met over 200 representatives of national and local organisations in round-table discussions and talked, in their homes or places of work, to many people who had been directly affected. Finally, we invited over 100 people to be interviewed. Everyone has been willing to help. This is my chance to place on record my thanks and appreciation to all who contributed. I have special reasons to thank my secretariat team who laboured so willingly, often in trying circumstances. I would also like to thank those officials in The Netherlands, France and at the European Commission in Brussels who gave up their time to meet us and answer our questions.

This Inquiry set out to address the major features that characterised the handling of the epidemic. Throughout the course of our work we were informed of many events specific to one location or even to one individual's experience. I particularly want to thank the many hundreds of people who took the time to share with us their first-hand accounts of what happened, thereby contributing to our knowledge. Because a particular story is not referred to in the report does not mean it has not influenced our thinking. Indeed, our understanding of what happened has been built up layer by layer from all the information we have collected.

My job was not to write a comprehensive history of the epidemic. Nor was it to conduct research into the mass of veterinary and epidemiological data that now exists. That said, and precisely because I do not want the rich vein of material we have assembled to be lost, I decided to publish (on CD-ROM and the Internet) the submissions along with notes of interviews. The only small exceptions to this are where members of the public have written to us on condition that we do not publish their statement or where we had purely informal exchanges, for example, in farmhouse kitchens. It is, I believe, very important that all the relevant scientific data collected by DEFRA during the epidemic is published quickly. This will allow further detailed research to be carried out.

It is worth repeating here that I was asked to conduct a completely independent inquiry into the Government's handing of the epidemic. Those who peruse the summary and then the detail of the Inquiry's findings will discover that a number of constructive criticisms are made. Here, though, I should like to air some personal observations which should be seen in the light of the overall analysis contained in the report itself.

History repeats itself

We seem destined to repeat the mistakes of history. In the Northumberland Report of 1968, and back through the decades, similar conclusions to ours were drawn about the need for preparation, the rapid deployment of resources and the central importance of speed, above all speed-to-slaughter of infected animals. The epidemic of 2001 presented unprecedented challenges which no-one in any country had anticipated. But better preparation to support speedier deployment of critical skills and faster action on the ground to slaughter infected animals and their close contacts would have limited the scale of the damage.

Immediately prior to this outbreak, contingency plans were in place. But maintaining and updating these plans was not a priority at national level. If the best preparatory work found in some locations had been replicated nationally, the outcome for the country as a whole would have been better.

Although Ministers and their veterinary experts and officials recognised from the outset that they were facing a serious situation, no-one in command understood in sufficient detail what was happening on the ground during these early days. We examine in the report both the reasons for this lack of detailed intelligence and its consequences, as well as making recommendations.

In government, departmental responsibilities are paramount. On day one MAFF recognised its responsibility, as did all other departments. MAFF was in charge. This meant that the wider resources of government were not mobilised early on. Ministers who were dependent on complex veterinary and official advice were expected to answer to Parliament with confidence and clarity. At the same time they were expected, via the media, to give reassurance to the public that what needed to be done was indeed being done.

Confidence gives way to panic

The truth started to emerge in early to mid-March. Some relationships among those involved became tense. A sense of panic appeared, communications became erratic and orderly processes started to break down. Decision making became haphazard and messy, not least in the way in which the culling policy was to be extended. The loss of public confidence and the media's need for a story started to drive the agenda.

For those of us outside the machinery of central government, it may be hard to appreciate the difficulties faced by Ministers and officials at such times. They are constantly in the front line. Yet they are tightly constrained, their every word closely monitored and analysed. This is an important aspect of 'lessons to be learned'. The normal processes of government need to be adjusted to handle an emerging national crisis effectively. Government has already recognised this challenge and has put in place a procedural and structural response system for dealing with it.

Management of the crisis

The process by which all the resources of government are put at the disposal of the centre of government is co-ordinated in the Cabinet Office Briefing Room (COBR). This specifies a set of procedures and structures designed to bring an orderly flow of decisions, resources and actions to bear on the management of a crisis. COBR has flexible design principles and may be led, as was the case for some time in this epidemic, by the Prime Minister, or by any Minister appointed by the Prime Minister. When it takes a decision, the government as a whole, with all its departments, stands committed to deliver on it.

The role of COBR is examined in more detail later in the report. It made a massive contribution to the way the epidemic was eventually brought to an end. It was convened 31 days after the first case was notified, by which time 479 cases had been confirmed.

Breakdown of trust

Whatever central government does and however well, it cannot defeat a major outbreak of animal disease on its own. It needs to co-ordinate the support and services of many others, including those most directly affected. This was the case throughout the epidemic of 2001 and will be so in any future outbreak. Wholehearted support for a common purpose depends on mutual trust and confidence. One finding of this Inquiry has been the extent of the breakdown of trust between many of those affected directly or indirectly and their Government. Many people have chosen to speak about this based on the experience of their own eyes and ears.

It is well beyond the remit of this Inquiry to speculate on the wider implications of this lack of trust and confidence. I simply say that success in the fight against any future major outbreak of animal disease will depend on the co-operation of farmers and many others in the countryside. It will also depend on farming and tourist interests recognising that they have a joint stake in the success of their rural communities. Similarly, central government must regain the confidence of, and work more in partnership with, local government.

The way ahead

During the course of the Inquiry we have been faced with criticism of the Government's policies and actions throughout the epidemic. I recognise the frustration and anger felt by so many. I understand the desire to see someone blamed. I also understand that, farmers in particular were subjected to stress and sometimes to insensitive behaviour on the part of officials. But, equally, I am satisfied that the officials I have met in Whitehall and in the regions were trying to cope in sometimes desperate, almost impossible, circumstances.

The nation will not be best served by seeking to blame individuals. Rather we should seek to apply the lessons to be learned in a manner that will contribute to changes in collective attitudes and approaches. In that way we can, in future, approach the shared task of being better prepared and better able to respond with speed and certainty.

Trust and confidence cannot be built by the independent actions of one side alone. DEFRA should take the lead, but others must follow. From the insights obtained throughout the Inquiry I have formed the opinion that a first step is for DEFRA simply to admit that government made mistakes during its handling of the crisis and that all involved are determined to learn from these mistakes.

Within MAFF, and now DEFRA, I detected a culture predisposed to decision taking by committee with an associated fear of personal risk taking. Such a climate does not encourage creative initiative. It inhibits adaptive behaviour, and organisational learning which, over time, lowers the quality of decisions taken. It seems to me that a reappraisal of prevailing attitudes and behaviours within the Department would be beneficial.

This report describes our understanding of what happened and why. It sets out the major lessons to be learned, together with a set of recommendations for action. I hope that not only the Government but everyone with an interest in the future of farming and the wider rural economy will look to learn these lessons, apply the recommendations and thereby collectively ensure that the experience of 2001 is never repeated.

Iain Anderson
July 2002

2 INTRODUCTION AND SUMMARY

Introduction

The Foot and Mouth Disease (FMD) epidemic of 2001 was one of the largest in history. Our Inquiry sets out the lessons to be learned from it and makes recommendations for action.

This is the report of one of three independent inquiries announced by the Government in August 2001. The Policy Commission on the Future of Farming and Food published its report in January 2002. The Royal Society published its report into infectious disease in livestock in July 2002. We have not sought to duplicate their work. Nor have we gone into detail on the financial aspects of the outbreak, which have been covered by the National Audit Office in its report published in June 2002.

It is worth making two points at the outset. First, given the wide spread of the disease throughout the country prior to detection, the impact of this outbreak was bound to be very severe. Even had everything been done perfectly by all those concerned to tackle the disease, the country would have had a major epidemic with massive consequences. Second, many farmers, local people and government officials made heroic efforts to fight the disease and limit its effects. Through their efforts it was finally overcome and eradicated after 221 days, one day less than the epidemic of 1967-68.

This report covers England, Scotland and Wales but not Northern Ireland. The following is a summary of our findings.

Summary

The last major epidemic of FMD in the UK was in 1967-68. Following that outbreak, the 1968 Northumberland Report made a number of recommendations for action, some of which were still relevant in 2001.

An outbreak of FMD was unexpected. Neither MAFF nor the farming industry was prepared for an outbreak on a large scale. The Ministry could not cope with the unprecedented chain of events which allowed the disease to go undetected for some weeks. However, in those areas where the number of cases remained low, disease control was more effective. Ultimately, the disease was contained and was prevented from becoming endemic.

A contingency plan was in place, and agreed by the European Union, but it had gaps and had not been shared widely or vigorously rehearsed outside the State Veterinary Service. The scale of the outbreak, and the way in which it spread, could not have been anticipated. The State Veterinary Service had, over the previous two years, expressed internal concerns about their readiness for an outbreak of FMD. These concerns were not relayed to Ministers. Warning signs, from the experience of classical swine fever in The Netherlands in 1997 and in Britain in 2000, were not acted upon. The country was not well prepared for what was about to unfold.

The first responses to the early cases were not fast enough or effectively co-ordinated. The paramount importance of speed, and especially the rapid slaughter of infected animals, was not given overriding priority early on.

Knowledge within government of some changes in farming and farm practices was limited. In particular, the nature and extent of sheep movements which contributed to the wide dispersal of the disease before its identification had not been fully recognised. Information systems were incomplete and had to be developed during the outbreak.

Initially the outbreak was treated as an agricultural issue. MAFF took the lead within government in managing the outbreak. Almost immediately they came under severe resource pressures. The impact of the disease, especially on tourism and the rural economy, was not recognised early on. Although supported by many at the time, with the benefit of hindsight, the widespread closure of footpaths, with no straightforward mechanism for reopening them, was a mistake.

The scarcity of resources was not only confined to vets. There were important gaps in managerial and logistical skills. The quality of communication was mixed. Mechanisms for joining up government were not brought into play from the start. As a result this put enormous pressure on MAFF. The State Veterinary Service tended to work in isolation. This may have contributed to the fact that initially the depth of the crisis was underestimated. People worked long and hard, under very difficult circumstances, to try to contain the disease and limit the consequences. Eventually the armed forces were deployed in support and made an impressive contribution, providing leadership, management and logistical skills.

In Scotland, with a different management structure and closer relationships between central government, local government and the farming industry, the outbreak was better managed. Contingency planning had been more systematic and the disease did not spread so far. Key problems were identified early and dealt with quickly. In Wales, the lack of devolved powers for animal disease control was a source of tension and resulted in blurred lines of communication, responsibility and accountability between the National Assembly for Wales and MAFF, now DEFRA.

Opening COBR towards the end of March and the personal intervention of the Prime Minister, were both pivotal in managing the crisis. They brought to bear the full weight of Government on tackling the disease. A few days later and 35 days into the crisis, a scientific advisory group gathered for the first time under the chairmanship of the Chief Scientific Adviser to the Government.

A network of Disease Control Centres was set up in those areas where the infection was at its worst. These Centres, each run by a senior Regional Operations Director, made major contributions to controlling the disease.

Because disease control policy had not been debated widely before the outbreak, arguments took place as the disease was raging. Changes, in particular to culling policy, were introduced at short notice. Often they were poorly communicated. Large parts of the farming and wider rural community became mistrustful of government. The public and the media – which had initially been broadly supportive of the Government's approach – turned against it. In particular, the policies of culling apparently healthy animals, within 3km of infected premises, or on contiguous premises, became very unpopular, despite their contribution to disease control. Management of carcass disposal was a major concern, particularly in the early days, but improved significantly after the armed forces became involved. However, the operation of the scheme for disposal on welfare grounds was poorly managed and costly.

The issue of vaccination assumed a high profile, not least in the media. However, by the time it was agreed that vaccination should be used to help control the disease in Cumbria, the disease had passed its peak. In the event it was not used, largely as a result of opposition by the farmers' unions and parts of the food industry.

As the disease declined, an exit strategy was developed. This included targeting resources to the areas of residual disease, coupled with a robust use of biosecurity and a programme of blood testing. The introduction of the autumn licensing scheme for animal movements caused considerable difficulties and hardship for farmers.

The overall costs of the outbreak were enormous, totalling over £8 billion. Millions of animals were slaughtered. Different sectors of the economy were affected in very different ways. Farmers were compensated for animals that were culled for disease control purposes and for welfare reasons. Rural and tourist businesses however received very little recompense. Farmers whose stock was not culled, but who were subject to strict movement controls, received no compensation at all. Systems for valuation had not been developed in advance of the outbreak.

Looking ahead, the processes of horizon scanning, contingency planning, rehearsal and learning from mistakes should become part of government routine. The creation of DEFRA which replaced MAFF after the General Election in June 2001, and brought together agricultural and rural issues, offers the opportunity for such developments to take place.

Good communications are vital to any organisation's business. For a Government in time of crisis they are critical. This requires accurate, up-to-date, well targeted and local communications systems, using the best technology available.

Our report contains a series of recommendations which, if acted upon, will help ensure that: the chances of exotic animal disease entering the country are reduced; the farming industry itself is less vulnerable to outbreaks of infectious animal diseases; and that, if such a disease does occur, the impact is minimised.

Our recommendations form an ambitious agenda. But, taken in conjunction with the programme set out by the Policy Commission on Farming and Food and underpinned by the recommendations of the Royal Society's scientific report, we believe that they offer the opportunity to transform and protect the rural and agricultural economies and communities of Britain.

3 LESSONS TO BE LEARNED

The FMD outbreak of 2001 had a profound impact on all those communities and individuals involved. Collective learning from such a massive experience can have great value if it is carefully analysed and then well used.

Perhaps the biggest lesson of all is that no amount of effort can eliminate the risk of damage from FMD. To reduce the risk of economic damage as far as possible, requires a range of co-ordinated actions by Government, the farming industry and others in the rural economy working together.

Drawing on the experiences of the 2001 outbreak we have identified a number of themes which need continuing attention. These are the major lessons to be learned:

- **Maintain vigilance** through international, national and local surveillance and reconnaissance.

- **Be prepared** with comprehensive contingency plans, building mutual trust and confidence through training and practice.

- **React with speed and certainty** to an emergency or escalating crisis by applying well-rehearsed crisis management procedures.

- **Explain policies, plans and practices** by communicating with all interested parties comprehensively, clearly and consistently in a transparent and open way.

- **Respect local knowledge** and delegate decisions wherever possible, without losing sight of the national strategy.

- **Apply risk assessment and cost benefit analysis** within an appropriate economic model.

- **Use data and information management systems** that conform to recognised good practice in support of intelligence gathering and decision making.

- **Have a legislative framework** that gives Government the powers needed to respond effectively to the emerging needs of a crisis.

- **Base policy decisions on best available science** and ensure that the processes for providing scientific advice are widely understood and trusted.

These lessons should be incorporated into a national strategy designed to:

- **Keep out infectious agents** of exotic disease.

- **Reduce livestock vulnerability** by reforms in industry practice.

- **Minimise the impact** of any outbreak.

4 RECOMMENDATIONS

Building on the lessons to be learned, our first and central recommendation is as follows:

> We recommend that the Government, led by DEFRA, should develop a national strategy for animal health and disease control positioned within the framework set out in the report of the Policy Commission on the Future of Farming and Food. This strategy should be developed in consultation and partnership with the farming industry and with representatives of the wider rural economy. The European Commission, the devolved administrations in Scotland and Wales, local authorities and other agencies of government should be involved in this process.

Throughout the report, we draw out a further 80 recommendations as they emerge from our analysis in support of this over-arching recommendation. This section pulls together those recommendations grouped thematically. Each recommendation is numbered and has a page reference. They fall into three broad areas:

Developing and maintaining a national strategy for disease avoidance and control.

- Strategy
- Legislation
- Vaccination
- Farming practices
- Veterinary matters
- Biosecurity
- Training
- Import controls

Developing and maintaining appropriate contingency plans and ensuring effective preparedness.

- Contingency planning
- Scientific advice
- Information
- Public health
- Slaughter and disposal
- Animal welfare
- Human resources

Managing an outbreak of disease.

- Crisis management
- Speed of response
- Diagnosis
- Role of the military
- Communications
- Management controls

Developing and maintaining a national strategy for disease avoidance and control.

Strategy

The following recommendations offer specific proposals in support of our central recommendation on strategy:

Accepted best practice in risk analysis should be used by DEFRA and others in developing livestock health and disease control strategies.
(9, p.38)

Cost-benefit analyses of FMD control strategies should be updated and maintained. These should be undertaken at both the UK and EU level.
(52, p.139)

Where the control of exotic animal diseases has wider economic or other implications, the Government should ensure that those consequences for the country as a whole are fully considered.
(32, p.86)

The interests of all sectors likely to bear the brunt of any costs should be properly represented and taken into account when designing policy options to control animal disease outbreaks.
(51, p.139)

Disease control policies should be developed in consultation with those local authorities responsible for implementing them.
(63, p.153)

Lessons learned should routinely be reviewed in the light of changing circumstances. Policies, plans and preparations should be adapted accordingly.
(2, p.25)

The Government should make explicit the extent to which the wider effects of disease control strategies have been identified, measured and taken into account in policy decisions.
(50, p.137)

The Government should publish a biennial report to the nation on the level of preparedness to tackle animal disease emergencies. The first report should be published in 2003 and include measures of achievement against goals.
(11, p.39)

The resources and research programmes of the Pirbright Laboratory should be fully integrated into the national strategy for animal disease control and budget provisions made accordingly.
(65, p.159)

In developing the surveillance strategy, there should be the widest possible involvement of those with a role to play in surveillance.
(67, p.160)

Legislation

The animal health legislative framework should be robust, unambiguous and fit for purpose. This was not the case during the 2001 epidemic.

The powers available in the Animal Health Act 1981 should be re-examined, possibly in the context of a wider review of animal health legislation, to remove any ambiguity over the legal basis for future disease control strategies.
(77, p.163)

Provision should be made for the possible application of pre-emptive culling policies, if justified by well-informed veterinary and scientific advice, and judged to be appropriate to the circumstances.
(38, p.99)

Vaccination

The country's options for disease control should be decided in advance of any future outbreak of infectious animal disease.

Our Inquiry has not explored in detail the scientific issues concerning FMD vaccination, which were a central part of the remit of the scientific inquiry conducted by the Royal Society. We have, however, formed a view that the option of vaccination should be a part of any future strategy for the control of FMD. There are hurdles to be overcome: the science is not yet clear enough; many farmers and farming organisations have expressed their opposition; there are concerns about consumer reaction; there are complex EU and international issues. All these must be tackled urgently. The UK Government should take the lead in the international debate. We are not arguing for routine preventative vaccination to be adopted but, in the event of an outbreak, emergency protective vaccination must be an option available for use whenever judged by the veterinary experts to be appropriate. All necessary work to prepare for such a possibility should be put in hand. This means that:

The Government should ensure that the option of vaccination forms part of any future strategy for the control of FMD.
(48, p.129)

The Government should establish a consensus on vaccination options for disease control in advance of an outbreak.
(47, p.129)

The State Veterinary Service should maintain the capability to vaccinate in the event of a future epidemic if the conditions are right.
(49, p.129)

Farming practices

The livestock farming industry and government should examine the opportunities to reduce the risk of disease by influencing farming practices. Throughout our report we have identified a number of specific proposals for government that will contribute to this:

The Government should retain the 20-day movement restrictions pending a detailed risk assessment and wide ranging cost-benefit analysis.
(78, p.164)

The Government should develop a comprehensive livestock tracing system using electronic tags to cover cattle, sheep and pigs, taking account of developments at EU level. The Government should seek to lead the debate in Europe on this issue.
(79, p.164)

The UK prohibition of swill feeding of catering waste containing meat products should continue. The UK should continue to support a ban at EU level.
(15, p.49)

The Government should build an up-to-date database of livestock, farming and marketing practices. This should include research to examine the evolution of regional livestock stocking densities and implications for disease risk and control.
(5, p.30)

However, the Government can only do so much to prevent a recurrence of disease. The farming industry itself has a crucial role to play. We endorse the recommendations of the Policy Commission on the Future of Farming and Food on assurance schemes and recommend further that:

The livestock industry should work with Government to undertake a thorough review of the assurance and licensing options to identify those arrangements most likely to reward good practice and take-up of training, and how such a new system might be implemented.
(76, p.162)

Farm assurance schemes should take account of animal health and welfare, biosecurity, food safety and environmental issues.
(75, p.162)

We also urge the livestock industry, and its representative organisations, to do everything in their power to promote good practice, to tackle shortcomings and poor standards of farming, and to work within the framework of recommendations we have set out to reduce the risk posed by infectious animal diseases.

Veterinary matters

The State Veterinary Service provides the backbone for a national livestock health and disease control strategy. Maintaining a strong State Veterinary Service, at the centre of a surveillance and disease control strategy, and involving many veterinary and other agencies, should be a high priority.

Notwithstanding some of the proposals made to us, we do not support the devolution of State Veterinary Service responsibilities to Scotland. There are advantages in retaining an integrated organisation for Great Britain, not least in terms of national disease control strategies. However, we recommend the following:

As many functions of the State Veterinary Service as possible should be relocated from London to regional centres, particularly to Scotland and Wales.
(70, p.161)

There should be a reappraisal of Local Veterinary Inspectors' roles and conditions.
(3, p.28)

The Government should develop opportunities for increased use of veterinary 'paramedics'.
(69, p.160)

Biosecurity

Biosecurity measures must be a part of generally recognised good practice for everyone involved in producing and handling livestock. In the event of a serious disease outbreak good biosecurity becomes critical and should be enforceable.

Farmers, vets and others involved in the livestock industry should have access to training in biosecurity measures. Such training should form an integral part of courses at agricultural colleges.
(60, p.148)

The livestock industry and government jointly should develop codes of good practice on biosecurity. They should explore ways to communicate effectively with all practitioners and how incentives might be used to raise standards.
(61, p.150)

Training

During our Inquiry, gaps in people's knowledge and understanding of the factors involved in preventing and managing infectious diseases of livestock were brought to our attention. Filling these gaps is a long-term challenge for the industry, the veterinary profession as well as training centres, colleges and universities.

The Government should support a national action group charged with the responsibility of producing a plan to tackle the gaps in practitioners' knowledge of preventing and managing infectious diseases of livestock. To be effective this will need a timetable, milestones for achievement and incentives.
(71, p.161)

Colleges, universities and training organisations should provide courses to equip those working in the food and livestock industries, and those owning susceptible animals, with the skills and knowledge to enable them to recognise the signs of animal disease early and take appropriate action to prevent its spread.
(72, p.161)

Training for Local Veterinary Inspectors in exotic diseases should be intensified, and consolidated into ongoing training strategies.
(74, p.162)

DEFRA should commission a handbook for farmers on identifying and responding to animal disease, drawing on the experience of 2001.
(73, p.162)

Training for those responsible for managing disease control should include the relevant legal frameworks and the structure and responsibilities of local government.
(43, p.112)

DEFRA and the Department for Education and Skills jointly should explore with the veterinary professional bodies and higher education institutions the scope for increasing the capacity of undergraduate and postgraduate veterinary provision. Equivalent work should be done in Scotland and Wales.
(68, p.160)

Imports

The national strategy for livestock disease control must ensure that proper steps are taken to minimise the risk of incursion from illegal imports of meat and meat products. We recommend that:

DEFRA should be given responsibility for co-ordinating all the activities of Government to step up efforts to keep illegal meat imports out of the country. This should include better regulations and improved surveillance on illegal imports of meat and meat products.
(14, p.48)

The Government should ensure that best practice from import regimes elsewhere be incorporated with domestic practices where appropriate.
(12, p.47)

The European Commission should lead a targeted risk based approach designed to keep FMD out of EU Member States. The UK should work alongside other EU Member States to highlight areas of greatest risk.
(13, p.47)

The UK should urge the OIE to consider the implications, for the detection and control of FMD, of the removal of swine vesicular disease from the List A of notifiable diseases.
(64, p.156)

Developing and maintaining appropriate contingency plans and ensuring effective preparedness.

Contingency planning

DEFRA should develop further its interim plan, published in March 2002, in full consultation with all interested parties. Its relevance should be maintained through agreed programmes of rehearsal, practice, review and reporting. This work should be given priority for funding.
(81, p.165)

The following recommendations offer specific proposals in support:

As part of its contingency planning, DEFRA, the Scottish Executive and the National Assembly for Wales, working with the Civil Contingencies Secretariat, should examine the practicality of establishing a national volunteer reserve trained and informed to respond immediately to an outbreak of infectious animal disease.
(30, p.82)

Contingency plans should set out procedures to be followed in the event that an emergency expands beyond worst-case expectations.
(6, p.36)

Government departments should ensure that their own internal departmental arrangements properly resource contingency planning work. This should be monitored by the National Audit Office.
(10, p.39)

The contingency plans of DEFRA, the Scottish Executive and the National Assembly for Wales should specify the measures needed during an epidemic to monitor progress and report to key stakeholders.
(22, p.73)

The State Veterinary Service, together with the Pirbright Laboratory, should increase their horizon scanning and threat assessment capabilities for major infectious animal diseases.
(66, p.160)

The Government should build into contingency plans the capacity and processes to scale up communications systems and resources rapidly at the onset of any future outbreak of animal disease.
(53, p.142)

Where regional boundaries of Government Offices do not match those of local authorities or other agencies of government, special provision should be made in contingency planning for management and communications during a crisis.
(4, p.28)

The Restricted Infected Area ('Blue Box' Biosecurity arrangements) procedures should be built into contingency plans.
(62, p.151)

The National Assembly for Wales and DEFRA should develop a comprehensive agreement for co-ordinating the management of outbreaks of infectious animal diseases in Wales. This should cover all aspects of a disease outbreak, delegating responsibility locally, where appropriate, and providing clear lines of communication and accountability.
(31, p.84)

Scientific advice

The involvement of independent sources of scientific advice early in the 2001 epidemic was due to the personal intervention of the Chairman of the Food Standards Agency. The formal engagement of a scientific advisory group was not until 35 days after the start of the epidemic. In order to ensure the fullest access to best scientific and veterinary advice, we recommend that:

DEFRA's Chief Scientist should maintain a properly constituted standing committee ready to advise in an emergency on scientific aspects of disease control. The role of this group should include advising on horizon scanning and emerging risks. Particular attention should be given to the recommendations on the use of scientific advisory committees in The BSE Inquiry report of 2000.
(34, p.91)

Public health

FMD itself poses no risk to public health, but activities involved in managing an epidemic may create issues of public health concern. This was the case during the outbreak of 2001. We recommend that:

All agencies with responsibility for public health should be actively involved in designing disease control strategies and in contingency planning and communications.
(44, p.112)

Information

Without access to timely, high quality information decision-makers are handicapped. The FMD crisis revealed shortcomings in the information gathering and processing infrastructure. We recommend that:

DEFRA should lay out milestones for investment and achievement for improved management information systems.
(20, p.73)

Data capture and management information systems should be kept up to date and reflect best practice.
(21, p.73)

Standard definitions of all important parameters of information should be agreed in advance.
(23, p.73)

DEFRA's Geographical Information System and the Integrated Administration and Control System (IACS) should be designed so that they can be used more effectively for disease control purposes.
(19, p.72)

Use should be made of alternative sources of information and intelligence during crises.
(18, p.71)

Slaughter and disposal

Mass pyres and huge burial sites, used to dispose of the remains of millions of slaughtered animals, remain vivid images of the 2001 epidemic. We recommend that:

Burning animals on mass pyres should not be used again as a strategy for disposal.
(42, p.108)

DEFRA should revise its guidance and instructions for slaughter.
(28, p.78)

Local communities should be consulted on mass disposal according to best practice guidelines, and the question of compensation for communities accommodating emergency disposal sites be researched. We recognise that this is a complex legal area nationally and at EU level.
(45, p.114)

Animal welfare

One lesson from the experience of 2001 was that animal welfare cases rise rapidly during the course of an expanding epidemic. This may be the case in any major outbreak. We recommend therefore that:

The Government should consider the welfare implications of disease control policies, as part of contingency planning for FMD and other diseases, and should seek to identify strategies that minimise the need for slaughter and disposal on welfare grounds.
(46, p.119)

The joint DEFRA Industry Working Group for Animal Disease Insurance should ensure that its scope and membership is set widely enough to address valuation and compensation issues highlighted by the 2001 outbreak. Clear deadlines should be set for reporting progress.
(80, p.165)

Human resources

One of the biggest challenges in crisis management is to ensure that the right people with the right resources are in the right places at the right time. A strategy for personnel management during a crisis should be worked out in advance and kept up-to-date in collaboration with stakeholders. We recommend that:

DEFRA should develop its human resources plans for use in emergency. In particular they should focus on how staff numbers and expertise can be rapidly increased at a time of crisis. This should be developed in England in consultation with the Cabinet Office, the Regional Co-ordination Unit and the network of Government Offices. Similar arrangements should be developed in Scotland and Wales.
(8, p.36)

Contingency plans at regional level should include mechanisms for making effective use of local voluntary resources.
(24, p.74)

Contingency plans should provide for early appointment of Regional Operations Directors or their equivalent to take on operational management of a crisis. There should be a cadre of senior managers – not all of whom need come from central government – who can fulfil the role of the Regional Operations Director in an emergency and who should be trained in advance.
(33, p.87)

Managing an outbreak of disease

Crisis management

With the benefit of hindsight, there were insufficiently sensitive triggers in place to set off crisis warnings early enough.

There should be a mechanism, put in place at the centre of government, to assess potential domestic civil threats and emergencies and provide advice to the Prime Minister on when to trigger the wider response of Government.
(39, p.102)

The practice of crisis management was supported by the creation of the Joint Co-ordination Centre in Page Street. This influential group of senior officials, vets and military officers was joined by a representative of the National Farmers' Union and shared in the decision making and subsequent communication processes. This added value and we support this approach for the future. We recommend that:

A representative of the wider rural economy should be invited to participate in the Joint Co-ordination Centre.
(40, p.106)

At the height of the crisis the overall direction of policy and operations benefited from the direct involvement of the Prime Minister as well as senior ministers and officials. This meant that there was no senior group within government offering informed, but detached, advice that could challenge prevailing thinking. We recommend therefore that:

The concept of a 'senatorial group' should be developed to provide independent advice to the Prime Minister and Cabinet during national crises.
(41, p.107)

Steps should always be taken to explain the rationale of policies on the ground, particularly where implementation is likely to be controversial. Wherever possible, local circumstances should be taken into account without undermining the overall strategy.
(37, p.98)

Speed of initial response

In an emergency, such as an outbreak of FMD, it is important to react with speed and certainty, taking decisions and mobilising the required resources as soon as possible. A few hours gained or lost at the early stages can make a big difference. Preparation for rapid response is an important element of contingency planning. We recommend therefore that:

Provision should be made in contingency plans for rapid prioritisation of a department's work in the face of a crisis, and for speedy reassignment of resources.
(7, p.36)

In all suspected cases of FMD, the response should reflect the experience of the emergency services, where speed and urgency of action govern decision making.
(16, p.61)

The State Veterinary Service should consider forming a national network of 'flying squad' teams capable of responding to an alert. The continuing occurrence of false alarms can then be used constructively to maintain readiness and to practice routines.
(17, p.61)

Diagnosis

All the evidence we have received supports the need for more reliable and speedy diagnosis of disease. Modern diagnostic technology should be harnessed to contribute to the goal of acting with speed and certainty. We recommend that:

The State Veterinary Service should be routinely equipped with the most up-to-date diagnostic tools for use in clinical practice, to contribute to speed and certainty of action at critical times.
(36, p.95)

Role of the military

The contribution of the armed forces during the FMD crisis received much praise. The military can bring professional expertise and advice in managing an emergency. In particular, they have valuable logistical and operational management skills. However, since no two crises will be the same and, since the armed forces have their own priorities, it would not be possible or wise to make specific recommendations for the future based on their assumed availability. We do, however, recommend that:

As part of the mechanisms to trigger the wider Government response, the military should be consulted at the earliest appropriate opportunity to provide advice and consider the nature of possible support.
(29, p.82)

Communications

To have any chance of communicating successfully to all stakeholders it is essential to plan in advance.

A government-wide crisis communication strategy should be developed by the Civil Contingencies Secretariat with specific plans being prepared at departmental level; for example by DEFRA and the devolved administrations in Scotland and Wales in the context of animal disease control.
(54, p.142)

The Scottish Executive and the National Assembly for Wales handle communications separately. The following are recommendations to DEFRA. In Scotland and Wales we urge that systems should be reviewed as necessary to ensure equivalent standards are met.

We recommend that:

DEFRA should develop its regional communication strategy and ensure that it has effective systems for disseminating clear and concise information quickly to all its regional offices. This should be developed in the context of cross-government crisis management planning, in consultation with the Regional Co-ordination Unit and Government Offices.
(55, p.143)

DEFRA should resource its website to ensure it is a state-of-the-art operation. In any future outbreak, the website should be used extensively and a central priority should be to ensure that it contains timely and up-to-date information at national and local level.
(56, p.144)

DEFRA should commission research into the effectiveness of its direct communications during the Foot and Mouth Disease outbreak of 2001 so that all the lessons may be learned, acted upon and the results published.
(57, p.144)

The State Veterinary Service should revise all its disease control forms A-E and information about exotic animal diseases in liaison with the Plain English Campaign.
(58, p.145)

Communications strategies during a crisis should take special account of the needs of the international media.
(59, p.147)

Management controls

At the height of a crisis, the pressure to get things done may mean that proper management controls are overlooked. The National Audit Office examined this issue in its report of the FMD outbreak of 2001. We have a number of recommendations to add, from the perspective, of our own Inquiry, namely:

Dedicated control systems should be ready for use in a sustained emergency, and regularly tested as part of the contingency planning process.
(25, p.74)

The processes for procuring and delivering the necessary goods and services from external sources during a crisis should be reviewed. Systems should be tested to ensure they can cope with unexpected increased demands.
(26, p.74)

Priority should be given to recruiting accounting and procurement professionals to operate in emergency control centres during a crisis.
(27, p.74)

From day one of an outbreak, provision should be made to keep a record of all decisions made and any actions to be taken.
(35, p.93)

5.1 Introduction

Around mid-morning on Monday 19 February 2001, Donald Vidgeon, a drover of long experience, alerted Craig Kirby, the resident vet at Cheale's Abattoir in Brentwood, Essex to a problem with a batch of sows held over from Friday's shift. Mr Kirby examined the animals and saw how serious the problem was. Clinical signs alone can not distinguish swine vesicular disease from FMD. Both are notifiable diseases. He assumed, even hoped it was swine vesicular disease. First he stopped the production line. Then he telephoned the local office of the State Veterinary Service. About an hour later, after inspection by two government vets, one of whom had experience of FMD in Greece, there was no doubt. This was either swine vesicular disease or FMD. Only laboratory work could tell which.

This encounter, within sight of London's eastern skyline, signalled the start of the FMD epidemic that spread across Britain. By the end of September over 2000 premises had been declared infected, millions of animals destroyed and many rural lives and livelihoods affected in a manner unknown for a generation.

On that Monday morning none of the vets involved guessed that the virus was already incubating in more than 50 locations from Devon in the south to Dumfries and Galloway in the north. A rare set of circumstances had already determined that this would be one of the worst epidemics of FMD the modern world has ever seen. Numbers alone cannot capture the sense of what unfolded. The great epidemic of 2001 left an indelible mark on communities, businesses and people from all walks of life.

5.2 History

FMD was not a new phenomenon. Nor were the techniques for controlling it. On the face of it, an outbreak in 2001 should have been controllable using conventional strategies. These include the slaughter of infected animals and 'dangerous contact' animals (so-called 'stamping out'). Such methods had been used effectively in the isolated FMD outbreak on the Isle of Wight in 1981, and they worked in 2001 in those parts of the country where the number of cases was small and resources were not overwhelmed.

The outbreak in 2001, however, was far from conventional. The way in which the disease had spread before its discovery and had disproportionately affected sheep were both unprecedented. The failure to tackle the disease quickly by traditional methods led to alternative culling approaches being adopted. These are discussed in section 10.

Different livestock diseases have different economic impacts which change over time and vary from country to country. In Britain, throughout the early part of the 19th century, no attempt was made to eradicate FMD. Compared with other animal diseases, such as cattle plague, its symptoms

were relatively mild and mortality rates low. Yet, by the end of the 19th century, perceptions of the importance of FMD had changed. It became a notifiable disease, despite farmers opposition.

Legislation originally passed in the 1880s allowed for slaughter, with compensation, of FMD-infected animals and their contacts. However, this was rarely invoked until the major epidemics of the early 1920s when all diseased and contact animals were slaughtered except for valuable pedigree herds. Since then, stamping out has been the preferred approach for controlling FMD in Britain.

The desire for a better understanding of FMD in order to improve control policy led to the creation of the Pirbright research facility in 1924. The Pirbright Laboratory, now part of the Institute for Animal Health, is the UK's centre of excellence in FMD research and is the World Reference Laboratory for FMD. We refer to it throughout this report as the Pirbright Laboratory.

On the continent, immunisation techniques were developed in the inter-war years but not used in Great Britain. A Government report after the major FMD outbreak in 1952-4 contained extensive discussion of vaccination. It concluded that stamping out remained the right policy for Great Britain in general, adding that "in the case of a severe epidemic" vaccination might be a valuable or even indispensable weapon.

By contrast, in other parts of Europe, vaccination was used both as a control mechanism to throw a ring around specific outbreaks and, routinely, along land frontiers.

Between 1922 and 1967 there were only two FMD-free years in the whole of Great Britain. Four epidemics were so severe that they prompted official Government reports in 1922, 1924, 1954 and 1968, the last conducted by Lord Northumberland and known as 'the Northumberland Report'.

There is a high degree of continuity in the central themes of these reports. Recurring issues include: the importance of contingency planning; the role and supply of vets; speed of response; the impact of animal movements; the use of swill as a source of infection; restrictions after markets; tagging of animals to aid identification; and liaison between central and local government.

All these issues featured in the 2001 outbreak. That is why we say that it is perhaps easier to identify lessons than to learn and act upon them.

5.3 The Northumberland Report

One of the constant refrains surrounding the 2001 outbreak is that the lessons of the Northumberland Report were not learned. The CD-ROM annexes contain a full list of the Northumberland Report's recommendations and a summary from DEFRA of the extent of implementation of each of them. Frequently, the recommendations relating to disposal of carcasses and the role of the military have triggered critical comment.

5.2.1 History repeats itself

"[The initial outbreaks] were followed by an unprecedented number of outbreaks which were reported at such a rate as to overwhelm the existing staff of the Ministry, and to necessitate the immediate recruitment of an emergency staff whose time was fully occupied in dealing with the cases as they arose."

Foot and Mouth Report, 1922

"During the whole of this time the movements of animals in the district had been proceeding unhindered – in fact with unusual expedition. Rumour – as has so often been the case – preceded action by responsible authorities; … there was a rush to move animals out of the district before the standstill restrictions normally imposed by the Ministry could become effective. Crewe market was carried on as usual and the animals exposed there were dispersed."

Foot and Mouth Report, 1924

"A single outbreak that was not reported early enough was responsible for half the outbreaks during the epidemic."

Foot and Mouth Report, 1954

"There is difficulty in recruiting veterinarians to the Veterinary Field Service of the Ministry of Agriculture and it is essential that the Ministry should attract a reasonable number of good veterinary graduates who will later be available for promotion to the important posts which carry responsibility for controlling animal diseases like foot-and-mouth disease. Satisfactory disease control depends on a strong State Veterinary Service."

"We have studied carefully the control procedures laid down by the Ministry of Agriculture and which have been put into operation in the past when outbreaks of the disease have occurred. We consider that these procedures in general have been satisfactory but were not adequate during this unprecedented epidemic. Our main recommendations and suggestions therefore relate to the need for more detailed pre-outbreak planning for the mobilisation of manpower and equipment to deal with an outbreak wherever it may occur."

Northumberland Report, 1968

On disposal, the Northumberland Report concluded that: *"burial of carcasses is preferable to burning"*. Off-farm and mass disposal were not discussed as they did not arise. In 2001, 48% of the 600,000 tonnes of carcasses generated by the outbreak, including welfare cases, were disposed of by on-farm burial and burning. A further 14% went to mass burial and 16% to commercial landfill. Scope for burial was constrained by an increased awareness of the potential contamination of groundwater. This was aggravated by very high groundwater levels during the wet winter and spring of 2001. Disposal issues are discussed further in section 12.

On the role of the military, the Northumberland Report stated: *"it appears that assistance from the Armed Services is normally available to Government Departments when all other suitable labour resources have been exhausted. ...There was no delay in or difficulty in obtaining Service assistance when the 1967/68 epidemic became widespread. ...speed and efficiency in slaughter of infected and in-contact animals, disposal of carcass and disinfection of premises are the most vital elements in controlling an outbreak and these will not be achieved without disciplined workers under experienced and trained supervisors. .... After the epidemic ... agreement was reached that, in FMD outbreaks, any of the Ministry's [of Agriculture] regional controllers could approach Army Commands for assistance as soon as they considered that all suitable civilian labour resources had been committed. We recommend that the approach should not be delayed; liaison should be established forthwith ... and be maintained"*.

The role of the military is discussed further in section 9. However, the links established with the armed forces after 1968 were not maintained. This was, in part at least, a result of the reduced size and changing nature and role of the armed forces since the mid sixties.

5.3.1 Military personnel 1967-2001		
1967	Military servicemen and women:	445,050
	Civilian support:	353,850
	Total:	**798,900**
2001	Military servicemen and women:	211,200
	Civilian support:	111,700
	Total:	**322,900**

The criticism that the Northumberland Report was not implemented is, inevitably, simplistic and generally not well-founded. Many of the Northumberland Inquiry's specific recommendations were, by 2001, simply overtaken by developments. For example, *"Exempting animals carried by rail through Infected Areas from restrictions provided they are not untrucked"* has limited relevance today. Equally, constitutional developments, most notably the UK's membership of the European Union have profoundly changed the legislative and trading framework.

Nevertheless, some of Northumberland's recommendations have stood the test of time and would have helped in the fight against the 2001 outbreak. The Northumberland Report attached great importance to *"the early*

recognition of the disease and immediate action in stamping it out"
and to *"measures designed to limit the spread by controlling movements".*
It also emphasised that *"control procedures should be based on veterinary considerations only and should give rise to as little disturbance of normal commercial and public activities as such considerations would allow".*
And its main recommendations and suggestions related: *"to the need for more detailed pre-outbreak planning for the mobilisation of manpower and equipment to deal with an outbreak wherever it may occur."*

Despite the similarities, comparing 1967 with 2001 is not always fruitful. Ministry and veterinary structures have changed considerably over the past thirty years, as has the social, economic and political landscape. Contingency plans had not kept pace with changes in society.

2. We recommend that lessons learned routinely be reviewed in the light of changing circumstances. Policies, plans and preparations should be adapted accordingly.

5.4 Changes 1967-2001

Since the last significant FMD epidemic occurred in 1967, we have chosen that as a useful reference year for comparison with the present day. The most fundamental differences between 1967 and 2001 are the UK's membership of the EU, coupled with structural change in livestock farming and a reduction in its relative economic importance and profitability (5.4.2). In parallel with these changes there has been a growth of rural leisure and tourism.

Agriculture has become increasingly regionalised over the period with livestock concentrated in the North and West and arable farming in the East. Land tenure arrangements have led to far greater fragmentation of farm holdings, with farmers often keeping livestock on land widely scattered from the farmstead itself.

Similarly, the State Veterinary Service has changed since 1967 (5.4.3).

5.4.1 Local and Temporary Veterinary Inspectors

Local Veterinary Inspectors are mainly private practice veterinarians who are appointed by Ministers as agents to carry out certain areas of work on behalf of the Department. Local Veterinary Inspectors are appointed to specific panels, eg. TB, brucellosis, anthrax, export of horses etc. They can only carry out work for the panel to which they are appointed and for which they are trained. In 2001 there were approximately 7,000 Local Veterinary Inspectors.

Temporary Veterinary Inspectors are registered veterinary surgeons who are appointed on a temporary basis to the State Veterinary Service. There were 117 Temporary Veterinary Inspectors routinely employed by the State Veterinary Service prior to the outbreak.

The impact of change on veterinary surveillance and response

The number of vets employed by the State and its agencies in 2001 was roughly two thirds that in 1967. The most sizeable reduction in the State Veterinary Service was in the number of vets in middle management roles. Reliable data are difficult to obtain. DEFRA's own figures show that front line veterinary officer numbers fell from around 270 in 1967 to 220 in 2001. Moreover, problems of veterinary recruitment in the South East, mean that the State Veterinary Service headquarters is currently operating with 10 of its 27 posts vacant.

The changes to the State Veterinary Service stemmed in part from a reduction in the volume of work required as farming and animal health practices evolved, although recent events, including BSE and the pet passport scheme for rabies, have driven the workload back up without a matching increase in resources.

5.4.2 Changes in the farming economy 1967-2001

	Immediately prior to 1967/68 outbreak	Immediately prior to 2001 outbreak
Policy Context	Pre Common Agricultural Policy; UK market still open to significant imports of food.	Period of Common Agricultural Policy reform and re-opening of EU markets to significant imports of food.
Economic performance (livestock and dairy) England Output per £100 input	£114–117 depending on sector.	£75-94 depending on sector.
Average size of dairy herd England & Wales (Proportion over 100)	30 (12%)	76 (55%)
Average size of flock of breeding ewes England & Wales (Proportion over 500)	131 (25%)	267 (56%)
Annual UK slaughter of prime cattle	2.5-3.0 million	2.2 million
Annual UK slaughter of sheep	12-12.5 million	18 million
Annual UK slaughter of pigs	12.1-13.4 million	12.6 million
Proportion of meat retailed by independent butchers (GB)	83%	12.5%
UK self-sufficiency in beef	72%	100% plus
UK self-sufficiency in sheepmeat	36%	95%
UK self-sufficiency in bacon and ham	42%	50%
UK self-sufficiency in pork	96%	100% plus
Number of auction markets in England and Wales	380	180
Number of abattoirs in Great Britain	2,200	360
Approximate number of farm holdings in England	260,000	146,000

The changes also reflect a shift away from direct government delivery of services to greater use of agencies and privately contracted work. A 1995 review of the State Veterinary Service recognised the need for a balance to be struck between these elements. Although much of the State Veterinary Service work could, in theory, be removed from central Government control, there was a need to retain the capacity to respond to an animal health emergency.

We conclude, from the data above and from the views submitted to us by vets with many years experience, that insufficient attention was given to the relationship between the core State Veterinary Service and other parts of the veterinary surveillance and response network, including the private practice veterinary sector. The economics of farming mean that vets are

5.4.3 The State Veterinary Service 1967-2001

Year	State Veterinary Service	Agencies	SVS numbers	Notes
1967	Included Central Veterinary Laboratory, a laboratory in Scotland, Cattle Breeding Station, and Veterinary Inspection Service.	n/a	not known – approx 600	Animal Health Divisional Offices 26 in England 5 in Wales 19 in Scotland
1971	Agricultural Development & Advisory Service created, incorporating State Veterinary Service.	–	–	–
1979 –1980		–	597	Review of MAFF structures.
1986	Agricultural Development & Advisory Service became a charging organisation, State Veterinary Service reintegrated into the Ministry.	–	just over 500	–
1987		–	–	Animal Health Divisional Offices reduced to 44.
1990	Veterinary Inspection Service reviewed – reduced to 5 Veterinary Investigation Centres England/Wales, 8 in Scotland.	Central Veterinary Laboratory and Veterinary Medicine Directorate became agencies.	430	–
1993-1995	Moratorium on recruitment to State Veterinary Service.	–	–	–
1995	Review of MAFF Animal Health and Veterinary Group implemented.	Veterinary Inspection Service merged with the Central Veterinary Laboratory to become the Veterinary Laboratories Agency. Meat Hygiene Service created – 12 vets transferred.	just over 300	Animal Health Divisional Offices 15 in England 3 in Wales 5 in Scotland
2001		Veterinary Laboratories Agency employed 99 vets Meat Hygiene Service employed 40 permanent vets and 5 casuals, with 462 contract vets also on the books.	286 (220 in the field service)	Approx 100 Temporary Veterinary Inspectors employed in normal times. Some 7,000 Local Veterinary Inspectors also formed part of the veterinary network.

less likely to be called out to animals today than they were in 1967. At the present time there is less extensive routine surveillance and fewer large animal veterinary practices from which to draw vets in a crisis.

The Local Veterinary Inspector arrangements, which the British Veterinary Association reported to us as dating back to 1937, had not been reviewed and updated to meet changed circumstances. The Department had planned discussions with the Association on Local Veterinary Inspector appointment and training in February 2001. The first meeting had to be cancelled because of FMD. Discussions have now recommenced. The question of veterinary capacity and surveillance is addressed in section 17.

3. We recommend that there be a reappraisal of Local Veterinary Inspectors' roles and conditions.

Regional and central government

The structure of UK regional and local government in 2001 is very different from that of 1967. In Scotland and Wales, devolved administrations now take many executive decisions. The Scottish Executive has sole policy responsibility for all, and the Welsh Assembly for many animal health matters within the context of the UK's EU obligations. In both Scotland and Wales, ministers are locally accountable for aspects of rural policy. In England the county structure and the two- and three-tier systems of local government are, in many parts of the country, far removed from the structure of the mid 1960s.

Central Government too has evolved. In 2001 the network of Government Offices for the Regions in England had an important role in co-ordinating the operation of Government policy in the regions. However, only some Departments were under their umbrella. MAFF only became part of the Government offices on 1 April 2001 and DEFRA remains part of that structure. In many parts of Great Britain, the regional boundaries of some of the many Government agencies responsible for responding to FMD did not match. This made management and communication more difficult.

4. We recommend that where regional boundaries of Government Offices do not match those of local authorities or other agencies of government, special provision be made in contingency planning for management and communications during a crisis.

Public opinion

Animal welfare issues have assumed a far greater importance in the public mind since 1967. Public confidence in farming, science and government was damaged by the BSE crisis. Contingency planning had not kept pace with these developments. There had been no recent public debate on slaughter and vaccination so key components of the disease control strategy lacked the backing of public consensus.

5.4.4 The European Union and disease control

In contrast to 1967, Community legislation now covers many areas of disease control and trade in animals and products of animal origin in Member States. These include: animal identification; health rules applicable to intra-community trade of most species of animals and their products; health rules applicable to imports from third countries of animals and their products; procedures for control of the list A diseases specified by the International Animal Health Organisation, the OIE (17.1.1); veterinary checks on animals and animal products which are traded; and notification of outbreaks of relevant diseases.

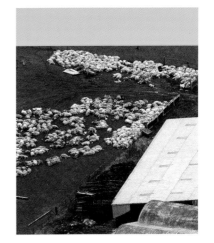

Directive 85/511/EEC, which came into force on 18 November 1985, provides for compulsory notification of suspicion of FMD in Member States. As soon as notification is made to the Commission, the holding is to be placed under official surveillance.

In addition, where disease is confirmed, all animals of susceptible species are to be slaughtered under official supervision. Carcasses of slaughtered animals must be destroyed in such a way as to prevent the spread of FMD virus. Meat, milk and milk products from the infected premises must be traced and destroyed, as must all substances likely to carry the virus. All farm buildings and equipment must be cleansed and disinfected.

At the same time that infection is confirmed, a Protection Zone of at least 3km radius and a Surveillance Zone of at least 10km radius from the infected premises is to be established.

Fifteen days after completing preliminary cleansing and disinfection of the infected holding, the rules in the Protection Zone are relaxed and the rules in the Surveillance Zone are applied instead. The Surveillance Zone restrictions may not be lifted for at least 30 days after cleansing and disinfection of the infected holding.

The Directive requires an inquiry to be carried out to establish the length of time the virus may have existed, the possible origin of the disease and its likely means of spread.

Disinfectants have to be approved by the competent authority and animals moved from their holding have to be identified.

Routine vaccination against FMD is prohibited but limited emergency vaccination is permitted under certain conditions.

The Commission is reviewing the existing Directive to take account of the 2001 FMD outbreak. Detailed proposals are expected later this year. The Commission is also working up new proposals on identification and traceability of sheep, including electronic tagging, as well as reviewing the import controls in place to protect the Community.

5.5 Sheep in the 2001 epidemic

A significant difference between the 1967 and 2001 outbreaks was the fact that, in 2001, sheep played a critical role. The 1967 outbreak was largely restricted to cattle and pigs. There were over 2,300 cases, confined mainly to cattle farming areas, in particular the North West Midlands and North Wales. The disease lasted 222 days and 434,000 cattle, pigs and sheep were slaughtered. The total number of animals slaughtered for disease control purposes in 2001 was more than ten times this, yet the 2001 outbreak comprised 2,026 cases. The reasons for this increased slaughter rate are discussed in section 10. A comparison of the 1967 and 2001 outbreaks is in the Appendix at 18.4.

In other outbreaks around the world, the predominant pattern has been for pigs, not sheep, to play a key role in spreading infection to cattle. There were almost 60% more sheep in England in 2001 than in 1967, concentrated in the northern parts of the country. The symptoms of FMD are not highly visible in sheep which is why the disease became widely disseminated before detection.

5. We recommend that the Government build an up-to-date database of livestock, farming and marketing practices. This should include research to examine the evolution of regional livestock stocking densities and implications for disease risk and control.

The wide dissemination of FMD in 2001 was exacerbated by the nationwide pattern of sheep movements throughout February 2001. This was due to the nature of sheep farming and, in part, to the agricultural changes referred to in section 5.4 above. Seasonal movement of sheep for fattening, in response to grass growth and climatic differences around the country, is long-standing practice. The distances involved have been great ever since the advent of transport by railway in the 19th century. The movement of sheep purchased by a dealer from Devon at the livestock market in Longtown, Cumbria, was a feature of the 2001 outbreak, but this was not a new phenomenon. Dealers have played a significant role in livestock markets for decades. There has been no collection of data on the extent of dealing activity over the years, so the significance of this part of the market is not well understood. Changes in the supply chain arising from the growth of supermarkets and the reduction in abattoirs may have increased the role of dealers in putting together batches of animals to meet demands.

Other developments that may have contributed to the scale of sheep movements in February 2001 include the Common Agricultural Policy annual premium which encourages farmers to ensure they have their full quota of sheep for the inspection period in February/March. MAFF was certainly aware of sheep movements but was taken by surprise by the volume of animals moving during February 2001. MAFF's initial estimate to Number 10 in the early days of the outbreak of one million movements was soon revised upwards to two million.

5.6 The run up to the 2001 epidemic

Before 2001, the continuing threat of BSE and the possibility of its appearance in sheep had been a major focus of activity for MAFF. It was unable to divert its scarce veterinary resources from this and other high profile investigations such as TB in cattle. For three months in the autumn of 2000, 80% of the State Veterinary Service resources had been absorbed dealing with the East Anglia outbreak of classical swine fever which comprised only 16 cases.

In 1997 in The Netherlands there had been a major epidemic of classical swine fever culminating in the slaughter of 9 million pigs. We have found no evidence of MAFF actively learning lessons from the Dutch experience, but we know that State Veterinary Service vets in the regions had acknowledged that they were poorly prepared for an exotic disease outbreak. Their concerns triggered an internal report into State Veterinary Service preparedness, the Drummond Report[1], written in 1999 (6.2).

5.7 The eve of confirmation

On the morning of 19 February 2001, when vets were called to look at some distressed pigs awaiting slaughter in Cheale's Abattoir in Essex, MAFF and the State Veterinary Service nationally had a number of top level priorities. Most prominent was the alarming possibility that BSE might infect sheep. There was also concern that classical swine fever might return and that scrapie in sheep could become extensive. The pet passport scheme and the control of rabies were high profile, as were problems with TB in cattle. There was concern too at the general level of resourcing of the service. Given these preoccupations among senior managers in the State Veterinary Service, the possible return of FMD, one of the most infectious animal diseases, was low on their list of priorities.

---

[1] Report of a Study of Notifiable Disease Preparedness Within the State Veterinary Service (Jan 1999)

6.1 Contingency planning

Contingency planning is the process by which organisations plan for uncertain events. Effective contingency planning covers all aspects of preparation for such eventualities, including: recruitment and training of staff; deployment of systems for administration and information management; installation of structures for management and decision making; sourcing of goods and services; and procedures for communicating internally and externally. A cornerstone of good contingency preparation is open communication among key partners to address strategies for response, including escalation, according to circumstances. Some organisations, notably the emergency services, have well-honed systems to respond to emergencies, and they rehearse and update them regularly.

The Government's Memorandum to our Inquiry stated that "comprehensive contingency plans were in place". We did not find this to be so. Papers laying out FMD contingency plans had been prepared and accepted by the European Commission and approved by the Standing Veterinary Committee. But we found the contingency plan limited in scope, out of date in some respects and not integrated into a national programme of rehearsal and testing. Some local government representatives and other stakeholders claimed they were not aware of these plans. One stakeholder referred to them as the "best kept national secret".

The contingency plans within MAFF consisted of three main parts: the plans submitted to the EU in accordance with Article 5 of Directive 90/423; the instructions issued to the State Veterinary Service for dealing with an FMD outbreak and contained in Chapter 3 of the State Veterinary Service's Veterinary Instructions, Procedures, and Emergency Routines (referred to in this report as the Veterinary Instructions); and the local Divisional plans drawn up by each Animal Health Divisional Office.

In March 1991, the European Commission published 'Recommendations or Guidelines for Contingency Plans against Foot and Mouth Disease DGVI/1324/9'. One of these recommendations was that each Member State should ensure that it had, immediately available, sufficient trained staff to deal with, at any one time, up to 10 cases and to maintain surveillance of premises in the 3km protection zone required around each. This was based on the scale of outbreaks previously experienced in Europe. A calculation made for the whole of the European Union during the preparation of Directive 90/423/EC estimated, in a worst-case scenario, 13 primary outbreaks, each with about 150 cases, throughout the Community over 10 years.

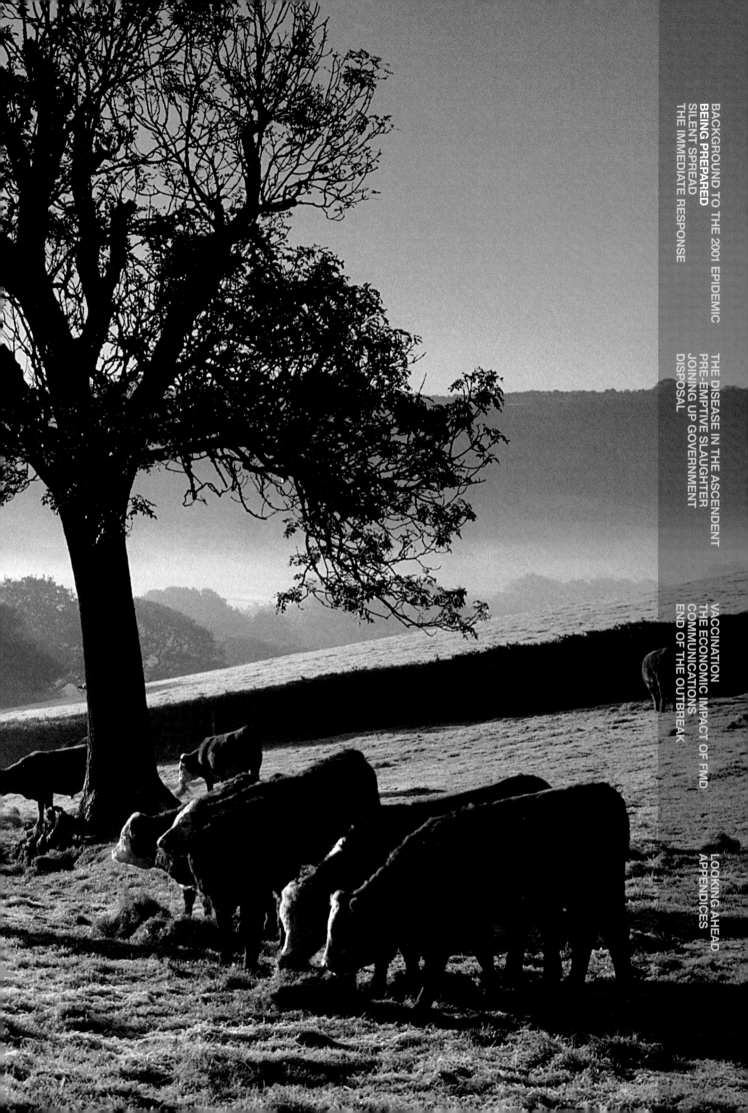

The contingency plan for Great Britain was approved by the Commission in 1993. This plan included the detailed veterinary instructions and guidance set out in Chapter 3 of the Veterinary Instructions. It described the legislative framework, financial provisions, national and local disease control centres, personnel resources, availability of diagnostic laboratories, epidemiologists and training exercises. Prior to the 2001 outbreak, the plan had last been updated in July 2000. It was not, at the time of the outbreak, available on the DEFRA website. It was placed there in August 2001.

The State Veterinary Service's Veterinary Instructions provide, in over 100 chapters, guidance and procedures for dealing with diseases and all the other tasks that the Veterinary Field Service performs. Chapter 3 which deals with FMD, is based on the EU agreed slaughter policy and disposal arrangements. This chapter provided the basis for managing the outbreak. Over 200 Emergency Instructions were issued during the outbreak. These reflected changes as policy developed and experience was gained in the field.

Each of the 23 Animal Health Divisional Offices is required to have contingency plans for FMD and other diseases. These plans were last checked and updated during 2000. They focused on ensuring that all the local information that might be needed in the event of an outbreak was readily available and that Animal Health Divisional Office staff knew how to implement the Veterinary Instructions.

6.2 The Drummond Working Group Report

In July 1998 the State Veterinary Service had been considering the state of its contingency planning. It set up a working group to study how well prepared it was for dealing with outbreaks of notifiable disease and to make recommendations for any necessary improvements. Richard Drummond, Head of the Veterinary Service in Harrogate, the lead region with responsibility for notifiable disease, chaired the working group.

His report, published in the CD-ROM annexes, was submitted in February 1999. It concluded that there was considerable variability throughout the State Veterinary Service in its readiness to deal with outbreaks of exotic, notifiable diseases. In particular, it was concerned about resources and identified five broad areas requiring action: training; contingency planning; infected premises work; use of information technology in outbreak control; and staffing and direction.

On contingency planning, it recommended that objectives and targets relevant to planning be included as work objectives within annual staff reporting. It urged that a template contingency plan be available on the MAFF Intranet, and that there should be increased awareness amongst the veterinary profession to the threat of notifiable disease. It also urged consideration to be given to the risks posed by the gathering of animals at markets, shows and large livestock units, and called for discussion of the ways in which contacts with local authorities could be established and best maintained.

In response to its own internal report, the State Veterinary Service agreed to target available resources to five priority areas. These were: making a generic emergency plan for FMD available for each Divisional Veterinary Manager to use if desired; formulating regional and Divisional training plans; preparing national guidance on overcoming the problems of supply of services and materials for dealing with outbreaks; ensuring up-to-date instructions were available for staff on-line; and discussing with the veterinary profession how to improve relations with Local Veterinary Inspectors.

In June 1999, the Chief Veterinary Officer emphasised the importance of emergency planning to deal with outbreaks of notifiable diseases. He acknowledged that resources had been concentrated on BSE, rather than on implementing the recommendations of the Drummond Report.

In July 2000 the Chief Veterinary Officer remained aware of the lack of progress on contingency planning. On 18 July 2000, the Assistant Chief Veterinary Officer in Wales wrote to the Chief Veterinary Officer expressing his concerns about lack of progress on implementing the Drummond Report recommendations, in particular those concerning the slaughter and disposal of carcasses and the training of staff.

The Chief Veterinary Officer was not only aware of the lack of contingency planning but had also visited the Pirbright Laboratory on 12 July 2000, where he was shown the deteriorating FMD situation in the Middle and Far East.

The Chief Veterinary Officer on 18 July 2000 wrote to colleagues within the State Veterinary Service expressing his concerns (in the CD-ROM annexes). However, his concerns were not exposed to Ministers or to the Department's Permanent Secretary. No action outside the State Veterinary Service was taken to tackle the significant shortcomings. We believe this contributed to a false sense of security within MAFF on 20 February 2001, when FMD was confirmed.

6.3 Weaknesses in the plan

It has been suggested to us that the level of preparation by MAFF was adequate for the generally accepted level of risk and that the extraordinary nature of this epidemic could not have been anticipated or prepared for. There is some truth in this argument. As noted above, the plan was based on EU guidelines suggesting that Member States should have the resources to deal with up to 10 simultaneously infected premises.

In developing its contingency plans, the State Veterinary Service used two scenarios – moderate and severe – each comprising 10 simultaneous outbreaks. The severe case scenario envisaged there being more premises at risk in the 3km protection zone around each outbreak. This would lead to a need for more tracings, including livestock movements through a market, than in the moderate case scenario. The severe case scenario

"Any contingency planning must be put in place which will identify the animals that are at risk of getting the disease and slaughter those animals only and not generate huge masses of carcasses which just puts intolerable pressure on any disposal system, whether it is rendering, incineration or whatever, because these animals shouldn't be in that processing system anyway."

*Public Meeting,
regional visit to the South West*

"May I pay tribute to the lay staff at MAFF Gloucester who played a large part in getting the right people to the right place at the right time. The veterinary team of three who planned action played their part magnificently, often working long hours. As a Temporary Veterinary Inspector I felt that I was most of the time being sensibly deployed. There seem to have been adequate staff for the jobs in hand. We were perhaps fortunate to have an influx of students at peak times and they worked hard and well."

Temporary Veterinary Inspector employed in Gloucester

"The whole organisation was sound asleep, they were asleep on their feet."

Public Meeting, regional visit to the North West

demonstrated that the UK would need 235 veterinary officers. The Commission judged the UK's readiness for disease outbreak as the best in the Community.

MAFF estimated that, in a more extensive outbreak, the number of staff needed might rise to 300. In such circumstances, it was expected that resources would be drawn from elsewhere within the service, the private sector and certain foreign countries with which agreements had been reached. *"…The State Veterinary Service did not often have to deal with crises on the scale of this FMD outbreak, and it had to come down to what was a reasonable insurance premium to pay in terms of maintaining high staff numbers…" (Senior MAFF Official).*

In the event, when FMD broke out, at least 57 premises were infected before the initial diagnosis was made. All State Veterinary Service resources were fully utilised almost immediately. During the course of the outbreak, over 2,500 Temporary Veterinary Inspectors were appointed, with nearly 70 from abroad. A further 700 foreign government vets and other secondees assisted on a temporary basis. There had been no assessment of the effects that a large-scale outbreak might have, or of how plans might be escalated. Better scenario planning would have left the State Veterinary Service more able to cope with the severity of the outbreak that it eventually faced. Planning should be comprehensive enough to deal explicitly with the challenges of scale-up. *"…The classical swine fever outbreak had stretched State Veterinary Service resources to their absolute limit so that when FMD struck it had, from the outset, rung alarm bells within the State Veterinary Service…" (Senior MAFF Official).*

6. We recommend that contingency plans set out procedures to be followed in the event that an emergency expands beyond worst-case expectations.

7. We recommend that provision be made in contingency plans for rapid prioritisation of a department's work in the face of a crisis, and for speedy reassignment of resources.

8. We recommend that DEFRA develop its human resources plans for use in emergency. In particular they should focus on how staff numbers and expertise can be rapidly increased at a time of crisis. This should be developed in England, in consultation with the Cabinet Office, the Regional Co-ordination Unit and the network of Government Offices. Similar arrangements should be developed in Scotland and Wales.

Contingency planning is not just producing a written document. Rather, it is about putting in place the systems, processes and culture to respond effectively to crises. Above all, it is about a shared sense of ownership and purpose across the relevant stakeholder community. We believe that the plans at national level would not have stood up to critical stakeholder scrutiny in advance of the outbreak. Deficiencies in critical resources could have been identified with prior communication and consultation.

6.3.1 Preparedness in Dumfries and Galloway

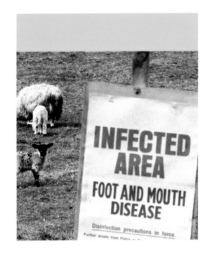

Dumfries and Galloway has a highly developed emergency planning approach – the Major Emergency Scheme – that has grown from its experience of the Lockerbie air disaster. This Scheme is based on a multi-agency partnership, co-ordinated by the Dumfries and Galloway Council.

Following activation of the Scheme on 28 February, the emergency planning group met daily throughout the outbreak and co-ordinated a wide range of support activities. These included: the establishment of the Emergency Room – known locally as 'the bunker'; local work to prevent spread of disease; setting up a logistics and transport operations centre; providing fully equipped accommodation centres for vets and military personnel; and establishing catering and welfare services.

As one submission commented, *"Contingency plans for the management of FMD are only as good as the working relationships between the organisations that are involved in the disease control campaign."* Co-ordination between the centre and local operations ensured that the policies determined by the Scottish Executive Environment and Rural Affairs Department, based in Edinburgh, were implemented effectively. The Scottish Executive Environment and Rural Affairs Department seconded staff to work with the Council and the Council was represented at relevant Scottish Executive committees. By contrast, MAFF did not fully exploit local authorities' expertise for management of emergencies in England.

The Council's Chief Executive and Emergency Planning Officer worked closely with the Regional Operations Director, the Divisional Veterinary Manager and Army Commander who jointly managed culling operations, once they were established in Dumfries. They met and updated each other at regular meetings, often two or three times a day.

Early and close involvement of the farming community contributed to the management effort. Unlike some areas in England, where the NFU felt marginalised, the NFU Scotland President was allocated space in the Scottish Executive Environment and Rural Affairs Department's Edinburgh offices.

The arrangements worked well. FMD was eradicated from the region within three months.

Time and again as we visited different parts of the country, at public meetings and in meetings with officials, we were given evidence of the limitations of the contingency plans that existed and of the wider community's lack of knowledge of these plans.

Coupled with this lack of consultation and awareness, the Inquiry also found that there had been little emphasis on training and simulation exercises. *"...In recent years there had been insufficient resources devoted to training, the rehearsing of contingency plans, and particularly I.T. systems because of competing priorities such as BSE..." (Senior MAFF Official).*

We found that some parts of the country were more prepared than others. In a number of regions rehearsals had taken place and internal lessons learned by the State Veterinary Service.

Staffordshire, for example, had been able to put its procedures and preparations to the test during the classical swine fever outbreak. Those involved believe that good communication at all levels and appropriate use of local knowledge were central to their ability to cope with the disease.

In Scotland, Dumfries and Galloway was also better prepared than most. The Scottish Executive in its submission acknowledged the impact that the experience of the Lockerbie air disaster in 1989 made on its contingency planning in that region. The local authority played a central role in managing the outbreak north of the border (6.3.1).

The best example of contingency planning that we identified was in The Netherlands. Prompted by the experience of a large outbreak of classical swine fever in 1997, the Dutch contingency plans had been thoroughly reviewed, tested, agreed with all key stakeholders and approved by Parliament before FMD appeared in Britain in February 2001.

6.4 Risk analysis

Contingency planning should not be seen in isolation. It is a dynamic process, not a static document. It must be linked into a wider process of risk analysis and disease prevention.

Risks should be managed so that the country can better respond to threats at an early stage. This can help to ensure that future animal disease emergencies are less likely to become crises, and that crises do not become disasters.

9. We recommend that accepted best practice in risk analysis be used by DEFRA and others in developing livestock health and disease control strategies.

6.5 Being better prepared

The contingency plans available in MAFF on 19 February 2001 to fight FMD met EU requirements but lacked scope. The plans that did exist were not widely exposed or rehearsed and, as a result, there was a limited shared sense of ownership by stakeholders. In addition, plans had failed to keep up with changing farming practices. Contingency planning was low down on the Department's list of priorities. It was not seen as part of a wider process of disease prevention and risk management.

10. We recommend that Government departments ensure that their own internal departmental arrangements properly resource contingency planning work. This should be monitored by the National Audit Office.

The eventual scale of the FMD outbreak could not have been foreseen. Nevertheless, better preparation, including better contingency plans, which were understood and well rehearsed would have done much to limit the scale of the crisis.

11. We recommend that the Government publish a biennial report to the nation on the level of preparedness to tackle animal disease emergencies. The first report should be published in 2003 and include measures of achievement against goals.

"Contingency planning, this should have been present already in view of the 1967 outbreak, the lesson should have been learnt then."

Public Meeting, regional visit to Wales

7.1 FMD and its virus

FMD is a highly infectious animal disease, caused by a virus. Its symptoms include lameness and lesions (blisters) on hooves and in or around the mouth. Signs of FMD are easily recognised in cattle and pigs. However, infected sheep often do not display symptoms and the disease can go unnoticed.

FMD does not usually cause death in livestock, except for young animals. However, contrary to the views of some it is not simply an equivalent of the common cold. Infected animals may suffer acute stress and pain. On recovery, their long-term health and condition may be affected, with serious economic impacts.

FMD spreads most effectively when susceptible animals are closely confined. Virus is present in the excretions, mostly faeces, and secretions such as milk, saliva and breath of infected animals. Animals become infected through inhalation or contact of the virus with mucosal membranes, especially in the mouth and nostrils.

Cattle and sheep are very susceptible to airborne virus, the former more so than the latter. Pigs are relatively resistant to airborne virus but very susceptible to contact infection, such as by eating infected feed. Infected pigs excrete large amounts of airborne virus – hundreds of times more than cattle – but cattle excrete the most virus in total, because they produce large amounts of infectious faeces and milk.

Airborne FMD virus can be carried great distances on wind plumes depending on weather conditions. For example, the 1981 FMD outbreak on the Isle of Wight was caused by a virus plume from Brittany, France. However, animals infected with the PanAsia strain of UK 2001 produced less airborne virus than other strains, so the potential for distant windborne spread was reduced.

Other susceptible species include goats, camels, llamas, deer and hedgehogs. Some, who attended the Inquiry public meetings, reported seeing wild deer display classical FMD symptoms and were concerned that they were spreading the disease. Although infected deer may transmit the disease, their living habits suggest that they are unlikely to have direct contact with livestock. Four hundred samples from deer were tested and all gave negative results. We believe that deer were unlikely to have spread FMD in this epidemic.

There are seven different forms, or serotypes, of FMD virus: types O, A, C, Asia 1, SAT 1, SAT 2 and SAT 3. Each serotype produces a distinct response in an animal's immune system, triggering a different set of antibodies. This means that, if an animal has immunity to a type A FMD virus, it may still be susceptible to FMD caused by a type O virus.

7.1.1 Relationship of FMD virus strains

Virus — FMD virus

Serotype — Type O   Type A   Type C   Asia 1   SAT 1   SAT 2   SAT 3

Strain — PanAsia strain

Isolate — UK 2001   South Africa 2000   Japan 2000

FMD viruses evolve, so that for each serotype, there are several different strains. Within those strains there are different sub-strains called 'isolates', which derive from individual outbreaks (7.1.1). The 2001 UK epidemic was caused by the PanAsia strain of FMD type O virus.

7.2 Global spread of the PanAsia O strain

The PanAsia strain has spread widely since its first appearance in India in 1990 (7.2.1). During the 1990s, it moved across the Middle East towards Europe reaching Greece in 1996. It also spread across Asia, causing several outbreaks in 1999 and 2000 in the Far East.

The PanAsia strain has never been identified in South America (7.2.2). Other FMD type O viruses have caused outbreaks there, but none was related to the PanAsia strain. Suggestions that FMD in the UK may have come from South America are therefore not valid.

In 2000, the PanAsia O strain took a major continental leap to South Africa. The incident was attributed to feeding pigs with untreated, infected meat from waste food. With hindsight, this should have been a warning that FMD remained a serious risk to any country, not just neighbours of those infected, especially through feeding swill to pigs.

The movements of the PanAsia strain and other variants of the virus before the UK outbreak were already well known to FMD experts. Predictions had been made that an epidemic of FMD was likely to hit Europe in the next few years. The European Commission for the Control of Foot and Mouth Disease convened an Expert Elicitation Workshop on the Risk of Introduction of FMD to Europe in September 2000[1]. The experts predicted that, within the next five years, one introduction of FMD was likely in each of the 'Islands' (UK and Scandinavian countries) and Western Europe groupings of countries.

[1] Estimating the risk of importation of foot-and-mouth disease into Europe. Gallagher et al. **Veterinary Record** (2002) 150, 769-772.

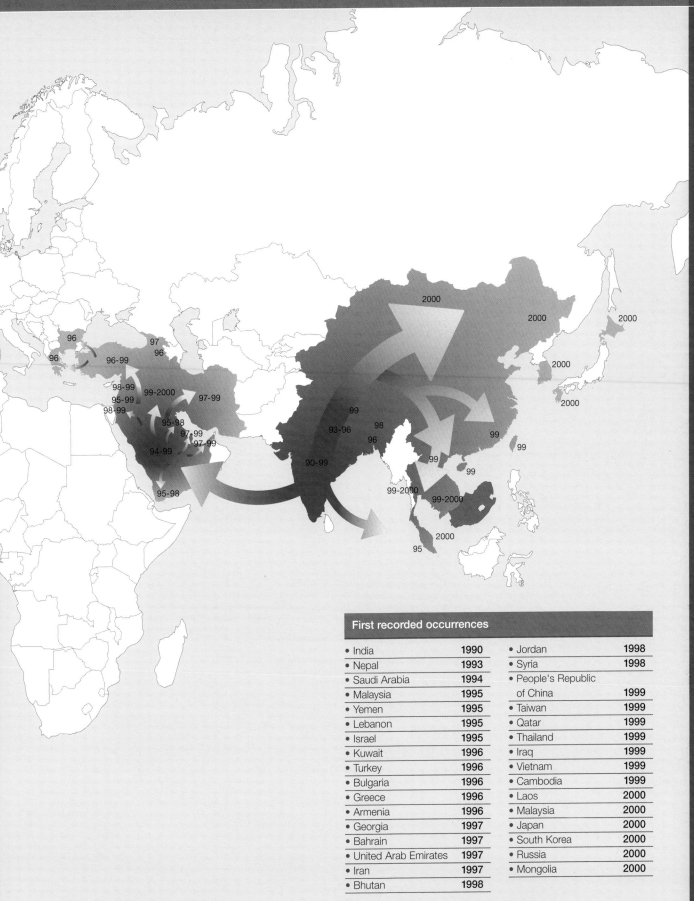

First recorded occurrences

• India	1990	• Jordan	1998
• Nepal	1993	• Syria	1998
• Saudi Arabia	1994	• People's Republic	
• Malaysia	1995	of China	1999
• Yemen	1995	• Taiwan	1999
• Lebanon	1995	• Qatar	1999
• Israel	1995	• Thailand	1999
• Kuwait	1996	• Iraq	1999
• Turkey	1996	• Vietnam	1999
• Bulgaria	1996	• Cambodia	1999
• Greece	1996	• Laos	2000
• Armenia	1996	• Malaysia	2000
• Georgia	1997	• Japan	2000
• Bahrain	1997	• South Korea	2000
• United Arab Emirates	1997	• Russia	2000
• Iran	1997	• Mongolia	2000
• Bhutan	1998		

Source: N.J. Knowles & A.R. Samuel, July 1999-May 2000 Institute for Animal Health
Pirbright Laboratory

7.2.2 Worldwide occurrence of FMD virus type O and the PanAsia O strain when first UK case confirmed

☐ PanAsia O strain
▦ FMD type O present

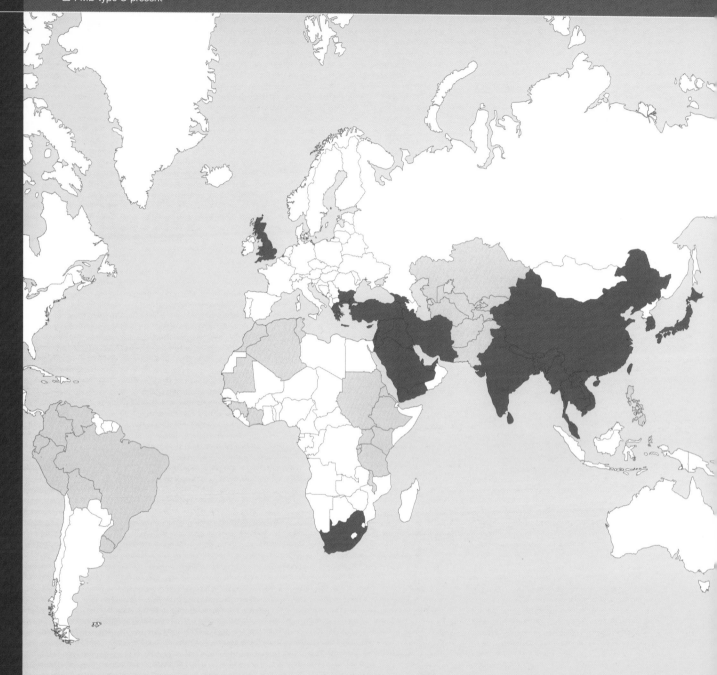

☐ PanAsia O strain
▦ FMD type O present

Source: Institute for Animal Health Pirbright Laboratory

Furthermore, the British Chief Veterinary Officer, Jim Scudamore, wrote to his deputies on 18 July 2000, saying, *"Having been at Pirbright for a day last week and seen the various maps of the deteriorating FMD situation in the Middle and Far East, there appears to be an increasing risk of incursions from exotic viruses."*

7.3 Entry of FMD into the UK

The exact source of the FMD virus implicated in the UK outbreak will never be known. Genetic analysis of the UK isolate showed that it bore the greatest similarity to the virus that caused the outbreak in South Africa in 2000. This information suggested that the two outbreaks were connected, either directly or by means of a common source. All the viruses which are most similar to these are from the Far East – the isolate from Japan 2000 being the most closely related. The UK and South African outbreaks both started through swill feeding of waste food. Although the possibility that FMD entered via imports from South Africa cannot be excluded, it is most likely that the source of FMD was a virus imported into the EU from the Far East[1].

7.4 The legal import regime

It is possible, but very unlikely, that the contaminated meat was legally imported. Legal imports have to be certified as originating in FMD-free countries or regions (7.4.1). Only de-boned matured beef is permitted to be imported from countries or regions that use routine FMD vaccinations. At certain temperatures, the FMD virus can live for at least five months in bone marrow and lymph nodes. Meat that has been de-boned and either heated to the centre to a temperature of at least 70°C or matured for nine months is considered to present negligible risks.

All meat consignments must be presented on arrival to a Border Inspection Post where they are subject to documentary and identity checks. At least 20% of consignments also undergo physical checks.

Legal imports have not taken place from any country where the PanAsia O strain of FMD occurs, apart from South Africa. On the basis of information available on imports, it is highly improbable that the disease could have been imported legally from South Africa.

Infected meat or meat products brought into the country as 'personal imports' are a possible source, but it is unlikely that these would enter the animal food chain. They are more likely to be consumed or discarded as domestic waste, rather than as catering waste that could be fed to livestock.

1 Origin of the UK Foot and Mouth Disease Epidemic in 2001, J M Scudamore, June 2002 in the CD-ROM annexes.

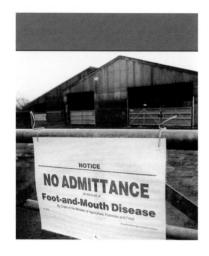

NOTICE
NO ADMITTANCE
on account of
Foot-and-Mouth Disease
By Order of the Minister of Agriculture, Fisheries and Food

7.4.1 Current import controls

EU legislation

Under the terms of the single European market in the veterinary sector, there are controls on the movements of animals and animal products into and within the European Community. The UK, along with all Member States, is subject to a system of veterinary inspection and certification.

Intra-community trade conditions

Animals and animal products imported into the UK from other Member States are not routinely inspected at the port or airport of arrival, but they are required to be checked at their premises of origin. Routine border checks on goods traded between EU Member States are not permitted. Random spot checks at the premises of destination are, however, permitted and determined by risk. The competent Authority in the exporting Member State is legally required to notify the receiving Member State of all consignments of live animals and some consignments of products (for example, raw material for processing) despatched. All imported live animals must have appropriate health certificates.

Personal imports from EU countries

Individuals are allowed to import meat, meat products, milk and milk products, other than raw, unpasteurised milk. Any individual attempting to import more than 10kg may be required to provide evidence that the commodities are solely for personal use. From time to time, further restrictions are introduced because of an outbreak of a specific disease in a certain country or countries.

Imports from countries outside the EU

As a rule, live animals or animal products imported into the Community may only originate from a country approved by the Community. The approval process takes into account such factors as the level of animal health in the country, with particular attention being paid to exotic animal diseases. Meat and meat products must originate from premises approved by the Community.

Commercial imports of livestock and animal products are only permitted into the EU through approved Border Inspection Posts. In Great Britain the State Veterinary Service and Port Health Authorities at seaports, and local authorities at airports are responsible for conducting veterinary and documentary checks on live animals and animal products imported from countries outside the EU through Border Inspection Posts.

7.4.1 Current import controls continued

Personal imports

Personal imports of meat and meat products from countries outside the European Community are prohibited, except for an allowance of 1kg of fully-cooked meat products that have been prepared in hermetically sealed containers.

The European Commission has recently come forward with a draft Regulation tightening rules on personal imports.

Waste food from ships or airlines could have been responsible for the outbreak. This material, which presents a high risk if fed to animals, was thought to be responsible for the outbreak of FMD PanAsia O strain in South Africa. EU and UK law prohibits the feeding of this waste food to animals. Food from ports and airports is collected under licence from DEFRA and destroyed by incineration or supervised landfill.

12. We recommend that the Government ensure that best practice from import regimes elsewhere be incorporated with domestic practices where appropriate.

13. We recommend that the European Commission lead a targeted risk based approach designed to keep FMD out of EU Member States. The UK should work alongside other EU Member States to highlight areas of greatest risk.

7.5 Illegal imports

Illegal shipments on a commercial scale are usually intended for wholesale outlets or for sale to restaurants or canteens. They are most likely to be illegally described or presented as non-food imports. This increases the chance of the virus getting into catering waste. If not properly cooked before feeding to livestock as swill, this material could reach pigs in sufficient quantities to cause disease.

The products that present the highest risk are those from regions where FMD is endemic. Meat, especially pork, still on the bone or with lymph glands attached, presents a serious risk as does de-boned frozen meat, especially pork. However, the likelihood of a significant quantity of frozen or chilled meat avoiding detection by Customs is low as it would tend to be transported using refrigerated containers and therefore easier to target.

Between 1 November 2000 and 9 April 2001, 1,321 Customs Declarations were selected as a control sample to test overall compliance with Customs requirements. All consignments selected were physically examined. None was found to have failed to declare meat imports.

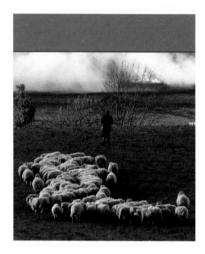

7.5.1 Import controls more strict in New Zealand than in the UK?

Many people have drawn comparisons between the import control regimes in the UK and several other countries. Perhaps the most common example brought to our attention was that of New Zealand.

New Zealand has a number of positive measures in place on personal imports, including a single biosecurity agency with a large presence at ports, supported by effective publicity, a system of signed declarations, amnesty bins for personal imports that break the rules, and on-the-spot fines.

Some of these measures may be suitable for the UK. However, it is important to take account of the practical circumstances that prevail in particular countries. New Zealand has 3.5m air passengers per year compared to 71m passengers arriving from outside the UK annually, of which 28m are from outside the EU. And New Zealand is a net exporter – 60% of its trade relies on agricultural exports. Maintaining low production costs is therefore economically critical given the distances to their markets.

Examining the policies adopted by other countries is a useful element in developing best practice at home. However, what is right for one country may not automatically be right for another. Even so, this caveat must not be put forward to justify any failure to adopt particular measures where they are both practical and effective.

It is difficult to assess the quantity of illegal meat that may be entering the country. However, the 2001 outbreak underlines the importance of continued vigilance by all authorities with border responsibilities in order to keep out the agents that can cause exotic infectious diseases.

DEFRA is leading interdepartmental consideration of the problem of illegally imported animal products (17.1). They may learn also from the control measures of other countries, such as New Zealand (7.5.1).

14. **We recommend that DEFRA be given responsibility for co-ordinating all the activities of Government to step up efforts to keep illegal meat imports out of the country. This should include better regulations and improved surveillance on illegal imports of meat and meat products.**

7.6 The spread of the disease prior to detection

Once the FMD virus had infected animals in the UK, the disease spread for weeks without detection. The probable timing of infection and transmission was judged by the age of the lesions on the animals inspected. Information about farms and movements of animals was used to trace the spread of the disease (7.6.1) (see CD-ROM annexes and Gibbens et al. paper[1]).

All the available evidence suggests that, sometime between mid-January and early February 2001, but most likely around 7 February 2001, pigs on Burnside Farm, Heddon-on-the-Wall became infected with FMD. Catering waste, containing illegally imported meat infected with the virus, is believed to have been fed to pigs as swill. By law, the swill should have been heat treated before use.

A ban on swill feeding was introduced on 24 May 2001. At that time, only 1.4% of the pig population in Great Britain were fed swill. Most domestic and catering waste was disposed of in licensed landfill. The additional volume generated by the ban was not considered to be significant.

15. We recommend that the UK prohibition of swill feeding of catering waste containing meat products continue. The UK should continue to support a ban at EU level.

The disease could have been present at Burnside Farm for weeks, but it went unreported, despite the requirement of farmers to report suspected cases of notifiable diseases.

Sheep and cattle on the nearby Prestwick Hall Farm, Ponteland, were the next victims of the disease. The farm is five kilometres north east of Burnside Farm and lies under the potential virus plume generated by the infected pigs. Weather conditions had been suitable for airborne spread throughout the likely period of infection. The most likely date of infection was 12 February 2001, although inspection of the animals suggested it might have occurred earlier.

FMD in sheep is difficult to diagnose. Farmers and vets can miss the signs. Infected sheep often display mild symptoms, if any, and suffer from other conditions that may be confused with FMD. Because cattle are more susceptible and show obvious signs of infection, they can act as sentinels for the disease, an 'early warning system'. The sheep on Prestwick Hall Farm were only diagnosed after the vet had been called out to inspect the cattle.

[1] Descriptive Epidemiology of the 2001 foot-and-mouth disease epidemic in Great Britain: the first five months. Gibbens et al. **Veterinary Record** (2001) 149, 720-743.

7.6.1 Probable initial spread of FMD

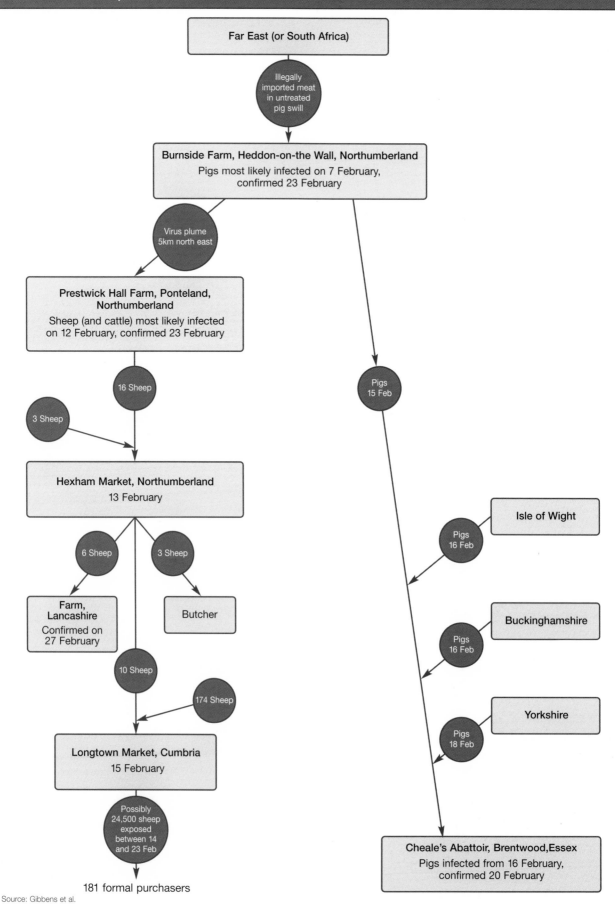

Far East (or South Africa)

Illegally imported meat in untreated pig swill

Burnside Farm, Heddon-on-the Wall, Northumberland
Pigs most likely infected on 7 February, confirmed 23 February

Virus plume 5km north east

Prestwick Hall Farm, Ponteland, Northumberland
Sheep (and cattle) most likely infected on 12 February, confirmed 23 February

16 Sheep

3 Sheep

Hexham Market, Northumberland
13 February

6 Sheep

3 Sheep

Farm, Lancashire
Confirmed on 27 February

Butcher

10 Sheep

174 Sheep

Longtown Market, Cumbria
15 February

Possibly 24,500 sheep exposed between 14 and 23 Feb

181 formal purchasers

Pigs 15 Feb

Isle of Wight

Pigs 16 Feb

Buckinghamshire

Pigs 16 Feb

Yorkshire

Pigs 18 Feb

Cheale's Abattoir, Brentwood, Essex
Pigs infected from 16 February, confirmed 20 February

Source: Gibbens et al.

Sixteen of these sheep went to market. On 13 February, together with three other sheep, they were sold at Hexham Market in Northumberland. Of the 19 sheep, three went to a butcher, six to a farm in Lancashire (which subsequently became an infected premises) and 10 to a dealer. The dealer took them to Longtown Market in Hexham on 15 February along with 174 other sheep. Potentially at least 24,500 sheep had passed through the market and been exposed to the disease between that date and 23 February when the movement standstill was introduced.

So, before anyone realised its existence, FMD had been seeded in many areas around the country. At least 57 farms in 16 counties were infected by the time the first case was confirmed.

Meanwhile, as FMD was spreading via sheep, infection had continued to rage on Burnside Farm. Infected pigs were sent to Cheale's Abattoir in Essex on 15 February and slaughtered on 16 February. Pigs that arrived at the abattoir on 16-18 February from the Isle of Wight, Buckinghamshire and Yorkshire, subsequently succumbed to the disease carried from Burnside Farm. Those animals were the first to be identified as suffering from FMD on 19 February.

7.7 Nature of the 2001 epidemic

Several conditions contributed to the introduction and widespread dissemination of FMD:

- The inclusion of infected meat in swill.
- The feeding of untreated swill to pigs.
- A delay in diagnosis of infected pigs.
- The infection of sheep by a virus plume.
- The undetected disease in sheep for weeks.
- Large number of sheep movements.

The nature of the 2001 epidemic was significantly different from the outbreak of 1967. In the latter, the disease affected mostly cattle, so diagnosis had been more straightforward. Most of the infection had been by airborne spread, though also through milk and animal movements. However, in 2001 the PanAsia strain was excreted in significantly lower amounts. So, airborne spread was not a major mechanism of transmission.

7.8 Alternative theories

During the outbreak, a large number of alternative explanations of the origin and mechanism of spread of the disease were put forward (7.8.1). Journalists who met the Inquiry told us that they investigated more than thirty such theories. Some of these ideas gained widespread popular support.

We have investigated a selection of these theories. In no case has the suspicion stood up to scrutiny.

"Had these sheep [from Longtown Market] been followed up and destroyed, and any other sheep they were in contact with had been destroyed immediately, those cluster bombs would not have been left there to manifest and go off and spread live virus all over the place."

Public Meeting, regional visit to Scotland

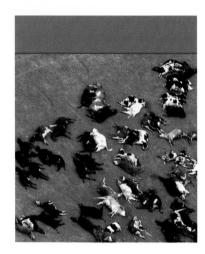

7.8.1 Alternative theories for the origin of the disease

Railway sleepers

One claim was that the Government knew that FMD was present in the UK long before February 2001 because MAFF had asked railway sleeper suppliers about their levels of stock shortly before the outbreak. DEFRA says that the enquiries were part of a routine exercise to update the lists of contractors identified in local contingency plans.

The enquiries in question were indeed standard practice. Lists of contractors from across the country, and details of the dates and locations of similar exercises, confirm this (see CD-ROM annexes).

Porton Down

In April 2001, a newspaper article claimed that live FMD virus had gone missing from the Government research facility at Porton Down and was used to start the outbreak deliberately.

None of the laboratories at Porton Down have either held live FMD virus before May 2001 or experienced any theft of microbiological material (see CD-ROM annexes). They could not have been the source of the outbreak.

Sheep exported to France

Positive test samples from sheep, exported from Wales on 31 January 2001 and arriving in France on 8 February, suggested that FMD had been in Wales in January 2001. When FMD broke out in the UK, the French authorities as a precaution culled all sheep imported from the UK from 1 February and took blood samples. In an initial virus neutralisation test carried out on this particular group of animals, seven out of thirty-one samples appeared positive.

We visited France and met the officials involved in these tests. They were absolutely clear that the first tests they carried out were false positives. When further tests were performed using protocols applied by other laboratories around the world, all samples gave negative results (see CD-ROM annexes).

Canada

In October 2001, a Sunday newspaper printed claims that the Canadian authorities knew that FMD was present in the UK in December 2000 and that travellers entering the country before Christmas 2000 had to wade through disinfectant baths.

A letter from the Canadian Chief Veterinary Officer states that these and other claims made in the article were "absolutely not true and without foundation" (see CD-ROM annexes).

7.8.1 Alternative theories for the origin of the disease
continued

Experimental farm

It is claimed that lambs infected with FMD were sold inadvertently from a Government experimental farm on the military range at Otterburn in Northumberland. The farm attempted to buy large number of lambs in a failed attempt to put the lid back on the disease.

The premises in question is the Redesdale experimental farm, run by ADAS Consulting Ltd. It has had no FMD-related activities. No FMD virus or vaccine has ever been kept there. And no livestock infected with, or vaccinated against, FMD has ever knowingly been kept on the farm. Inspection of the farm's livestock movement records since December 1999 revealed that no unusual movements of livestock either on or off the farm took place during the relevant period (see CD-ROM annexes).

8.1 The Abattoir

It was around 1030 on the morning of Monday 19 February, when Craig Kirby, the resident vet at Cheale's Abattoir, made his critical phone call to the local State Veterinary Service office in Chelmsford. Things at first moved quickly. Two state vets were despatched immediately to Cheale's, arriving shortly before noon. They both confirmed Kirby's initial suspicions. This was a classic case of either swine vesicular disease or FMD. Both are exotic viral diseases which may show indistinguishable clinical signs and symptoms. There was no doubt in any of the three vets' minds that this was definitely one of the two. Whichever it was, speed was of the essence.

A form A was issued declaring the abattoir an infected area. This meant that all movements in and out of the abattoir were stopped and tracing of all contacts was started.

An enormous amount of work was then needed at the abattoir to do a full clinical survey of all the animals. Advice on cleansing and disinfecting had to be given to all the people working there. Lorry loads of animals arriving in the afternoon had to be turned back

In accordance with their standing instructions, the vets took blood and tissue samples at around midday to send to the Pirbright Laboratory for immediate analysis. The vet from the State Veterinary Service phoned MAFF Head Office to explain her initial views. One of the Animal Health Officers from the MAFF local office drove the samples to Pirbright, around 70 miles away across London. The Animal Health Officer left Brentwood at around 1700 and arrived at the Pirbright Laboratory at 1900.

An email was sent from MAFF Head Office to the Pirbright Laboratory saying that the samples were on their way. In the event that email was never read, so the samples waited overnight at the Pirbright Laboratory before being collected the next morning. So, 12 hours of testing time had already been lost.

The first ELISA test to detect FMD (8.1.1) was started at 0900 on Tuesday 20 February. It was completed by 1330 and confirmed as a positive. MAFF was informed at 1350.

Back at the abattoir routine activity had ground to a halt. Work on slaughtering the pigs had been stopped as soon as the alarm was first raised on Monday. The process of culling infected animals under the supervision of the State Veterinary Service could not start without formal authority from Page Street.

By Tuesday morning, things had deteriorated. Many of the pigs were beginning to suffer extreme distress. Kirby himself authorised killing several of them on welfare grounds. Nothing further could be permitted until Pirbright scientists had completed their tests. After the first of these proved

8.1.1 Confirmation and diagnosis

FMD is confirmed primarily on clinical grounds. A vet needs to be convinced by the visible signs of the disease. Other than to confirm the first case of a new outbreak, laboratory diagnosis is only used for equivocal cases.

During the epidemic, there was significant confusion about whether laboratory confirmation was needed. Early on, MAFF Headquarters' staff at Page Street were not convinced by the telephone reports and instructed field vets to take samples. Lack of veterinary experience of FMD and the difficulty of diagnosing sheep which did not show obvious disease signs, led to a huge volume of testing.

Serious delays arose from waiting. Transport of the samples to the Pirbright Laboratory could take up to one day. Infected animals were to be slaughtered immediately after confirmation, but laboratory results could take four days.

Samples from animals suspected of FMD were tested for the presence of the FMD virus or specific antibodies which animals produce as part of their immune response to infection. Generally these antibodies can be detected from around five days after animals show signs of FMD.

The ELISA tests take about four hours, but the OIE 'gold standard' tests take longer. Virus isolation takes up to four days to confirm a negative, although positive results can be confirmed sooner. Virus neutralisation tests take at least two days.

Tissues likely to be infected, such as epithelium from lesions, are tested for virus by the direct sandwich (DS) ELISA and by the virus isolation test. The DS ELISA is also used to check that virus isolation positives are indeed FMD virus.

The liquid phase blocking (LPB) ELISA is used to screen blood samples for the presence of antibodies that recognise FMD virus. Positive or inconclusive samples are put through the virus neutralisation test.

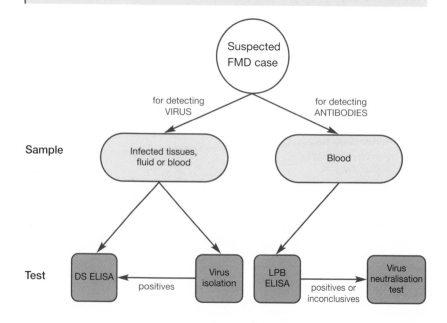

positive MAFF requested that a second be performed. That was completed later on Tuesday afternoon and it removed any remaining doubts. This was certainly FMD.

Even then the slaughter of all the affected pigs was not authorised. First, Dr Alex Donaldson, Head of the Pirbright Laboratory, needed to observe the clinical signs at first hand and collect samples. He arrived at the abattoir at about 1830 and confirmed classical symptoms of FMD in the pigs. He left at around 2000. The slaughter of the pigs began and was completed around 0100 on the following, Wednesday, morning.

By that time a farm next door to Cheale's Abattoir, had also been affected. This too was declared an infected premises, and slaughtering began there.

There are important lessons to be learned from the experience of those critical hours, from noon on 19 February until around 2000 on 20 February. That is why we have recorded in some detail what happened over that period of 30 hours. It is a time when speed can make such a precious difference. Standing Veterinary Instructions declare that, until laboratory tests are complete, a suspected case of swine vesicular disease should be treated as a case of FMD.

8.1.2 Slaughter of suspect pigs

The pigs at Cheale's abattoir were still alive several hours after FMD was first reported. Dr Donaldson of the Pirbright Laboratory has advised us that, in future, pigs with lesions should be slaughtered without delays and the carcasses kept for inspection, if necessary. The priority of slaughter should reflect those highest to lowest virus producers:

- pigs with generalised unruptured lesions;
- those with early developing lesions;
- those with ruptured lesions;
- the apparently healthy pigs.

With hindsight many things could have been done more quickly. Even without it, though, there are lessons that can be learned. During these precious 30 hours, the source of the infection could have been identified more quickly. Urgent phone calls could have been made to alert the Pirbright Laboratory to the samples on the way for analysis. The knowledge of Cheale's staff about the quality of the pigs received could have been sought. The expertise of their key staff would have offered at least a short list of possible sources. The Chief Veterinary Officer has told us that the records at the abattoir were hand-written and not easy to use. It took 48 hours to work through them all. Nevertheless, efficient record keeping, coupled with interviewing of the staff at Cheale's might well have indicated the index case more quickly.

By the evening of Tuesday 20 February, when the animals on the farm next to the abattoir showed clinical signs of FMD, there were at least three outbreaks of FMD in the country: one at the abattoir; one at the farm next door; and one or more other cases at a place or places then unknown, which had been the source of the virus reaching the abattoir.

At 0545 on the BBC's 'Farming Today' the next morning, Mr Ian Campbell of the National Pig Association said, *"The probability is that the infection... has actually occurred on contact in the abattoir and therefore it hasn't interfered with the vehicles that brought the pigs into that abattoir and infected these other pigs, but that is only a guess."* He also said, *"It's very serious and it requires every single pig producer in the UK to get straight out there and look at their stock and assess whether they have a problem... They should look very hard at their stock. They should identify anything which is out of the ordinary and showing lameness and immediately notify their vet for a double check to be made."*

The confirmation of FMD on 20 February led swiftly to a ban on exports on 21 February of live cattle, sheep, pigs and goats, and also of meat, meat products, milk and milk products and certain other products such as hides from these animals. But, apart from the strict controls around the places of infection, no animal movement restrictions were introduced across the country.

8.2 The ban on animal movements

Three days later, at 1700 on Friday 23 February, national movement restrictions were introduced. That morning an order was agreed by the Minister of Agriculture, after discussion with the Prime Minister, to come into force late in the afternoon. Animals in transit were allowed to complete their journeys. We were told by a number of people that the level of animal movements that evening was unprecedented.

The decision not to impose immediate movement restrictions was criticised time and again during our Inquiry. Are these criticisms justified? Once again hindsight can distort judgement. Even today the State Veterinary Service believes it would not have had the justification or the support to introduce widespread restrictions. Given the prevailing conditions we have sympathy for this view. Movement restrictions would probably have been seen as a disproportionate response. They would certainly have been very controversial. But it is an inescapable fact that the following could have been deduced by the evening of 20 February. Somewhere around the country, a pig farm was pumping out FMD virus and putting other farms and livestock at risk. Considering what is known about the infectious nature of this disease, we conclude that earlier movement restrictions would have been justified, and should have been ready to be put in place more quickly than they were.

Between 20 and 23 February the number of animal movements was substantial. The map of the animal movements (8.2.1) that did take place during those critical days shows just how great was the traffic.

△ Infected abattoir
▲ First case discovered
○ Infected farm or livestock dealer
◻ Index case

◻ Implicated market
➤ Movements on or before 20 February 2001
➤ Movements on 21 to 23 February 2001

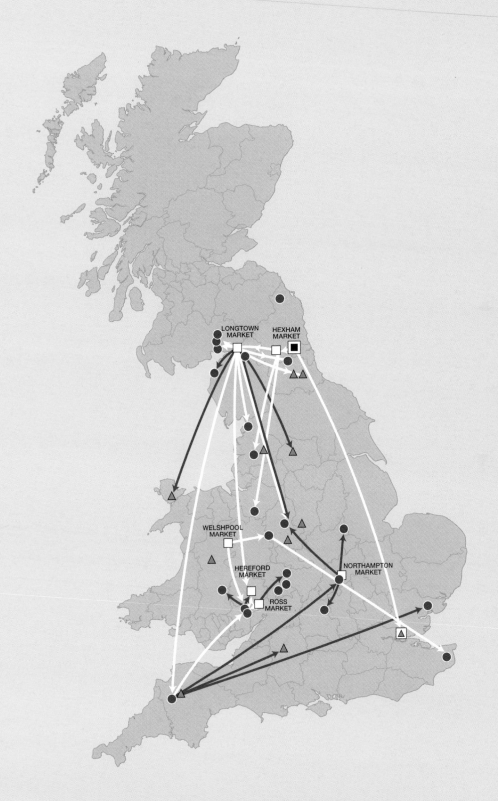

Source: Descriptive Epidemiology of the 2001 foot-and-mouth disease epidemic in Great Britain: the first five months. Gibbens et al. **Veterinary Record** (2001) 149, 720-743

Professor Woolhouse of Edinburgh University observed in evidence to the House of Commons Environment, Food and Rural Affairs Select Committee that:

"If we had imposed a national movement ban on 20 February, three days earlier, our estimation is that the epidemic would have been between one third and one half that it actually was."

Hours mattered. DEFRA epidemiologists have estimated that in the seven hours between the order having been signed and it coming into effect, 19 additional farms would have been infected – about three each hour.

In contrast, prompted by the knowledge of the outbreak in Essex, The Netherlands introduced restrictions on the transport of susceptible animals on 21 February. Precautionary action in Britain, similar to that carried out in The Netherlands would, without doubt, have reduced the size of the epidemic.

8.2.2 Tough decisions early on: the Dutch experience

A devastating outbreak of classical swine fever in 1997 had led The Netherlands to review thoroughly its contingency planning arrangements for dealing with major infectious animal diseases. The importance of speed of response had been one of the key lessons learnt from the Dutch experience and was a feature of their reaction to FMD in 2001.

After the first case of FMD had been confirmed in Essex on the evening of Tuesday 20 February 2001, The Netherlands imposed a transport ban the following day on all susceptible animals imported from the UK since 24 January 2001.

On the same day, a decision was taken to ban the collection of sheep within The Netherlands except for direct movements between farms or to slaughterhouses. Sheep movements to markets, collection centres, auctions and exhibitions were prohibited. This was extended to all susceptible animals on 22 February.

On 26 February, the transport of all sheep and goats in The Netherlands was banned, even to slaughterhouses. This was extended to all susceptible animals, following confirmation of the virus in France on 13 March.

Despite the swift imposition of these precautionary measures, The Netherlands recorded its first confirmed case of FMD on 21 March 2001. The source of the outbreak is thought to have been calves imported from Ireland that had come into contact with infected British sheep at a welfare staging point in Mayenne, France. This deduction was made only after confirmation of the first cases of FMD in The Netherlands, as the system for tracking animal movements between EU Member States did not record stops at staging points in third countries. The European Commission is reviewing the use of such staging points with a view to proposing further controls.

There is an overriding lesson to emerge from comparing the UK and Dutch experiences. It recurs throughout the story of the FMD crisis. The key to effective disease control is speed, speed and more speed.

16. We recommend that in all suspected cases of FMD, the response reflect the experience of the emergency services, where speed and urgency of action govern decision making.

Samples should be moved to the competent laboratory by the fastest means available. A senior member of the State Veterinary Service with appropriate clinical experience should be taken to the suspect site to determine and control the response, based on a risk assessment. Decisions should be communicated quickly at all times.

There are many unconfirmed cases every year and these should not generate a disproportionate response. Action taken should be in proportion to the level of risk. There should be a mechanism whereby, if experienced vets have no doubts about the presence of exotic disease, as happened with three vets on the morning of 19 February, a fast track procedure can be developed.

17. We recommend that the State Veterinary Service consider forming a national network of 'flying squad' teams capable of responding to an alert. The continuing occurrence of false alarms can then be used constructively to maintain readiness and to practise routines.

8.3 The Longtown connection

On Saturday 24 February, four days after the first case was confirmed in Essex, the first case occurred in Devon. The disease was identified on a sheep farm belonging to a sheep trader. He had bought sheep from Longtown market in Cumbria earlier that month. This batch had then been distributed to a number of different locations, especially in the South West of the country, many of which were eventually to succumb to the disease.

From this weekend onward the extent of the disease spread from Longtown became clear.

Some 25,000 sheep had passed through the market between 14 and 23 February, all of which could potentially have been exposed to FMD. They had then been dispersed widely spreading the disease silently before detection.

From 25 February, the MAFF epidemiological team began the work of tracing the sheep from Longtown. This was a slow task. With the head start that the disease already had, coupled with the enormity of the job in hand, MAFF was not well equipped to do it quickly. To complicate matters, there was the possibility that some dealing had taken place outside the market and there would be no record of those movements.

MAFF officials worked hard to trace all the contacts, but the process was slow. As late as 8 March they were still writing to farmers who had potentially bought sheep at Longtown. By then, the disease was widespread throughout the country.

8.4 Access: Footpath closure and its effects

In the early days of the epidemic there were understandable concerns that everything possible should be done to prevent the disease spreading. By the end of the first week and over that first weekend as the extent of the disease spread was becoming clearer, many people were urging more draconian measures, especially with regard to footpath closures.

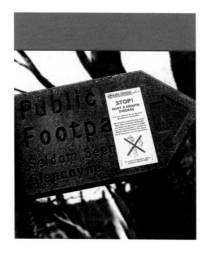

8.4.1 Footpaths

There are over 150,000 miles of Rights of Way in Great Britain. Local authorities are responsible for their management.

The powers to close footpaths in the context of an FMD outbreak stem from a Foot and Mouth Disease Order (1983) which reflected the views of the Northumberland Report. Under that order areas can be declared either 'infected' (areas of about 10km radius around infected premises) or 'controlled'. Controlled Areas were conceived originally as areas where temporary restrictions would apply pending the tracing of in-contact animals.

In Infected Areas the Order gives local authorities powers to close footpaths. A wide range of outdoor activities such as hunting, shooting and certain equestrian events are also prohibited. In Controlled Areas outdoor activities would normally be allowed with only deer hunting and stalking being prohibited.

In an unprecedented step the whole of Great Britain was declared a Controlled Area on 23 February 2001, and the associated restrictions lasted around nine months.

An amendment to the 1983 Order was made on 27 February with the intention of extending local authorities' powers to restrict access outside Infected Areas and to enable 'blanket closure'. Having been hurriedly introduced, the amendment did not provide the powers intended, so a second amendment was introduced on 2 March. Under this order, local authorities could close all paths within their boundaries without the need to place closure notices on individual footpaths. In areas where there were no cases of FMD, exercise of the powers was officially subject to clearance by the Minister. In practice local MAFF officials gave this clearance.

The power to impose new blanket closures was repealed on 16 March but existing closures were unaffected.

Some consideration was given to ministerial revocation of closure. In the context of impending local elections and expected opposition from farmers and some local councillors ministerial powers were not used.

In July 2001 the Minister revoked remaining blanket closures by declaration.

8.4.2 Closure of footpaths: different interpretations of the same thing

Official advice from MAFF was qualified. The first formal guidance to local authorities, in a circular dated 6 March, stated: *"[Power to restrict access outside Infected Areas] should only be used where there is evidence ... that to allow such unrestricted access would pose a potential risk of spreading the disease."*

The Prime Minister in his Internet broadcast on 27 February had said: *"...though we are not at direct risk from this disease, we can play a part, unknowingly, in spreading it. FMD is a highly infectious virus which can be picked up by us on our boots, clothes and cars and carried many miles. By staying away from farmland, by keeping off any footpaths through or next to farms or open land with livestock, we can help the efforts to eradicate this disease. We are giving local authorities today the power to enforce the temporary closure of footpaths and rights of way, but we hope people will voluntarily stay away in any case."*

In the House of Commons on 28 February, **Nick Brown, Minister for Agriculture**, said *"I deliberately left the issue to the discretion of local authorities, on the understanding that they would know best the local circumstances. It is for them to make an assessment of risk. ... Incidentally, if they want advice from me, I suggest that they act on a precautionary basis."* (Official Report col. 921) Later in the same debate, he said *"I urge local authorities to prosecute people who insist on arguing about those measures [to close paths]."* (Official Report col. 931)

NFU President Ben Gill on 27 February said: *"It is imperative that every local council which has rural footpaths and rights of way within its boundaries closes them immediately. There must be a blanket ban across the country. This could be crucial in helping us to stamp out this highly virulent disease. With new outbreaks being confirmed all the time, we are sure every responsible member of the public will support us. Remember the disease could be anywhere – not just in the restricted zones. I implore everyone once again: please, please stay away from the countryside."*

The NFU was calling for widespread closure. Other organisations supported the call for caution or took their own steps to close footpaths. On 22 February the Ramblers Association advised against taking rural walks. On 23 February the Royal Society for the Protection of Birds closed its nature reserves for a week. The National Trust announced the closure of all its parks containing livestock, and the British Mountaineering Council called on mountaineers and climbers to respect restrictions and stay out of the countryside.

No one knew where the disease might crop up next. By 26 February there were FMD cases in Essex, Northumbria, Devon, Wiltshire and Wales (Anglesey); by 27 February there were also cases in Northamptonshire, Durham and Lancashire.

The Government came under pressure from many quarters to extend the closure of footpaths and restrict access to the countryside beyond the official Infected Areas. MPs from all parties argued for temporary closure of rights of way in a debate on 26 February. The Welsh Assembly was concerned that the public were ignoring pleas to stay away from Snowdonia in particular. Officials in the Department of the Environment, Transport and the Regions were aware on 26 February that widespread closure would have implications for the whole rural economy, given that tourism is a larger rural business than agriculture. But they were sensitive to the wider mood of support for closures.

The Countryside Agency reported to us that, when they issued a press release on 2 March saying that costs to the rural economy could run to £2 billion, they experienced opposition from MAFF.

The audit trail for how the decision on footpath closures was finalised is unfortunately unclear (see recommendation 35 on page 93). What is apparent, is that following a series of meetings with the NFU and other stakeholders, and dialogue between MAFF and Number 10, Ministers sought powers to close rights of way beyond Infected Areas.

It is easy to understand the pressure Ministers were under to allow closure beyond just the Infected Areas. Many stakeholders were urging the Government to take action. They did so but not as far as we have been able to determine on the basis of explicit veterinary and scientific advice.

Many submissions stated that, with hindsight, this blanket closure of footpaths was mistaken. The National Trust described it as "the most costly decision of the entire outbreak", even though the Trust itself had initially supported closure.

Many tourist and leisure organisations realised quickly that the impact would be significant. As the realisation grew that the outbreak was unlikely to be short lived, many people began to recognise its potential impact.

The frequent changes in guidance, the lack of clarity in communication, the loss of confidence in the Government's scientific understanding and control of the outbreak, all hindered those seeking to get consensus on reopening. Farmers under tight biosecurity restrictions found it difficult to accept that walkers would not pose a risk. The public began to wonder why a disease that reportedly did not have much of an impact on animals and for which a vaccination was said to exist should be causing so much disruption. Only with the establishment of the Rural Task Force in mid March did a strategy begin to emerge for reopening footpaths based on a process of veterinary risk assessment. There was greater appreciation of the need to get the balance right between rural access and disease control. But, in terms of the wider economic impact on tourism and the rural economy, the damage had been done.

The decision on footpath closure contributed to the costs on the economy as a whole. Once this was recognised, the decision proved very difficult to undo since the reopening process had not been thought through at the time of closure. The role of local authorities was critical.

If future disease control measures necessitate the closure of footpaths local authorities, the National Parks and major landowners such as the National Trust should be consulted fully. The possibility of keeping livestock away from key heritage sites should at least be considered. This was suggested to us in the context of keeping open sites such as Hadrian's Wall to encourage continued tourism.

9.1 The national perspective

By 27 February, one week after the disease had been confirmed, a control strategy at a national level was in place. The initial policy response, of slaughtering all susceptible animals on infected premises and tracing and slaughtering dangerous contacts, had been put in hand, managed by the State Veterinary Service. These measures were supplemented by the nationwide ban on animal movements. On Tuesday 27 February, footpaths in all infected areas were closed and the Government empowered local authorities to close any footpath within their boundaries if they chose to do so.

This policy was in line with the pre-existing contingency plans, based as they were on the presumption of a relatively small, contained outbreak, the associated tracings of which could be completed reasonably quickly. What the policy did not, indeed could not, take into account was that the disease had remained undetected for three weeks during which it had spread throughout the country.

The advice that the State Veterinary Service gave to Ministers was that the policy would work. It was only a matter of time. This message was passed to Number 10 and the media.

On 21 February, Nick Brown, the Minister for Agriculture and Jim Scudamore, the Chief Veterinary Officer held the first of a series of daily press briefings on the state of the disease and the progress of the response, a development that was welcomed by the media. These briefings continued until 25 March.

The media's response to the disease in the first two weeks was broadly sympathetic. The view was that MAFF recognised the nature of the infection and the way it was spreading, as well as how to control and then eliminate it.

Other government departments were not greatly involved at this stage, largely because MAFF was not asking for help. However, on the first day of the outbreak, officials from the office of Baroness Hayman, a Minister at MAFF, contacted that of John Spellar, a Defence Minister, to raise the possibility that some form of military assistance might be needed if the disease could not be confined to one area.

The Cabinet Office carried out its traditional role of co-ordinating discussion across government. Over the following three weeks, official meetings were held to inform other departments of the impact of the disease and the measures being taking to control it. With the benefit of hindsight, there was much more that could have been done at this stage if information on the

actual state of the disease in the country had been available. For example, the Cabinet Office Briefing Room, known as COBR, which was to prove so effective in marshalling the full resources of Government to bear on the disease, might have been opened at this stage rather than 31 days into the crisis.

The outbreak was first discussed in Cabinet on 1 March. The minutes of that meeting indicate that the Minister of Agriculture gave a factual account of the disease control measures in place, which it was hoped would contain the spread of the disease. There was no discussion of the outbreak at the following week's Cabinet, due to the imminent budget. The next opportunity was the Cabinet of 14 March. By this stage, the impact on the tourist industry was becoming more apparent and was raised for the first time. On-site disposal was also discussed. The Minister reported that the priority remained to control and eliminate the disease. As yet he had not asked for any assistance from the Ministry of Defence other than to borrow veterinary officers.

At a national level, the shortage of qualified vets was the one real area of concern outside MAFF. The Chief Veterinary Officer wrote to his counterparts in Australia, New Zealand, Canada, USA and the Republic of Ireland on 23 February to request help. He followed this up on 25 February with letters to his opposite numbers in EU Member States.

Access to financial resources did not limit MAFF's response. The Treasury, in evidence to our Inquiry, told us that they had recognised at an early stage that disease control would cost more than MAFF's budget would allow. Aside from the need to ensure financial propriety and value for money, the Treasury placed no constraint on the resources available to tackle the outbreak.

MAFF experienced difficulty in converting offers of help from other government departments into practical reality. Promises of extra staff were sometimes not translated into action by those making them. And, where extra staff were made available, for example, additional press officers, the organisation was not in place to use them effectively. The Prime Minister helped address these difficulties by stating clearly that, whatever resources were needed to tackle the disease, should be made available. This was important, as it is extremely difficult to mobilise cross-government resources without such a clear statement of will from the highest level.

9.2 The view from the ground

However, at ground level, things were deteriorating.

On the weekend of 24-25 February the disease reached Devon. A vet there told us that he had been taking a walk on the beach with his family when he received confirmation of the first outbreak in the county. When he realised its location – at a farm belonging to a sheep trader – he said his heart sank. He decided to continue with the walk but told his family that they would not be seeing much of him for many weeks to come. Similarly, from a different perspective, the Head of Personnel within the State Veterinary Service told us that she recognised, during the same weekend of 24-25 February, that there was likely to be an "exponential" increase in the demand for vets and support staff.

Demands for manpower were indeed to grow exponentially. A single infected premises requires, as a minimum, a vet supported by a two-person team. After working at the infected farm, the team is classed as 'dirty' and has to be stood down for a period of time. The original infected premises generates a further set of farms to be traced and checked, each requiring yet another veterinary team. Meanwhile, in the early weeks of the outbreak, two or three other infected premises might be added each day. This typical scenario could increase the demand for field operatives very quickly indeed (9.2.1).

On Monday 26 February, once the first implications of the Longtown spread were becoming known and the first cases had been confirmed in the North East, leave for all State Veterinary Service vets was cancelled. The Prime Minister echoed the Chief Veterinary Officer's appeal for vets to volunteer.

Discussions took place about how to reduce vets' workloads to enable them to concentrate on core veterinary tasks and about how to allocate non-veterinary tasks to other staff. Some MAFF regional personnel were directed to support the immediate response. However, there were still too many non-veterinary tasks that, at this stage, had to be carried out by the most precious resource of all – the vets themselves.

By the beginning of March, there was a fast growing need for non-veterinary staff with a wide range of skills to which MAFF senior management was not sufficiently alert. The State Veterinary Service, particularly during the early stages, had tended to assert that it was "coping with the outbreak", and this was not challenged from the centre. As a result, no systematic effort was made early on to acquire additional, non-veterinary resources.

Part of the reason for this was cultural. The State Veterinary Service valued its independence and reflected this in its approach. There had been tension for many years within MAFF between administrators and vets, in general terms, no group would willingly choose to admit that it was not coping. Indeed, the State Veterinary Service may have felt that its successful handling of the classical swine fever outbreak of 2000 demonstrated that it could cope.

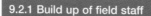

9.2.1 Build up of field staff

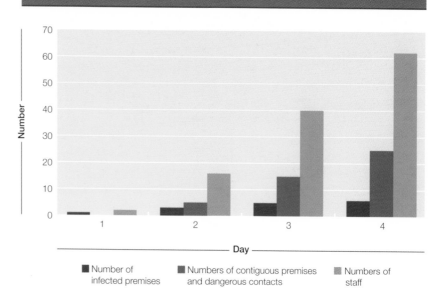

Day

■ Number of infected premises   ■ Numbers of contiguous premises and dangerous contacts   ■ Numbers of staff

Other activities expanding rapidly:

Slaughtermen
Vets/Animal Health Officers for surveillance
Foot patrols
Cleansing and disinfecting
Disposals
Licensing
Mapping
Epidemiology and tracings
Finance and contracting

Yet the warning signs of the fragility of the State Veterinary Service resources were there in 2000 and not picked up soon enough in 2001.

The Service was exhausted by the classical swine fever experience. Around 80% of its vets had been drawn on to tackle an outbreak that had consisted of just 16 cases. During the FMD outbreak that total was reached nationally on 27 February. By the end of the second week of the crisis, there were five times as many cases. The system was rapidly becoming overwhelmed. Clear messages about the severity of the worsening crisis were not getting through to senior management or Ministers.

At the same time, communications from senior management downwards also appeared to have difficulty reaching their target recipients. The message that FMD was an overriding priority did not filter through effectively to the rest of the Department. A human resources manager at DEFRA told us that the Department had a 'silo mentality' and individual groups and managers not directly involved with the outbreak remained focused on their own targets. There was no incentive for them to release staff to help in the fight against FMD.

It is a shortcoming that there was no inbuilt process for providing an alternative means of reconnaissance for MAFF's senior management.

Later in the crisis, the NFU played an important role in the Joint Co-ordination Centre by providing an additional source of information about what was happening on the ground.

18. **We recommend that use be made of alternative sources of information and intelligence during crises.**

Local police forces offered support, although there were differing views on what their role should be. For example, the police forces of Devon and Cornwall provided farm gate security at infected premises, viewing their role as one of reassuring and communicating with the local community. Avon and Somerset police, on the other hand, decided that a local security firm would handle this job better.

9.3 Management information systems

The situation was not helped by the difficulty in obtaining robust and reliable management data. It is impossible to tackle a crisis effectively without information about the developing situation and the performance of the emergency response measures. The management information systems available to MAFF at the start of the outbreak were not adequate.

The root of the problems can be traced back several years. The need for better use of information technology in disease control had been identified in the 1999 Drummond Report. Following the implementation of a major network solution in the early 1990s, staff had become increasingly comfortable with new technology. There was enthusiasm within the State Veterinary Service for applying new technology to disease control and planning.

However, in 1998, MAFF was set a budget that was seen as very tight. This came on top of a series of difficult spending settlements over a number of years. As a result, by the beginning of 2001, MAFF's computer systems had suffered protracted under-investment.

The earlier experience of dealing with classical swine fever had highlighted the importance of management information systems. However, development work had to compete for a limited pool of resources and made slow progress. When FMD broke out, MAFF's ability to record and analyse data about the spread and management of the disease was still based largely on a patchwork of unconnected systems operated by individual regions, some of which used only paper records.

To its credit, MAFF then moved quickly. On 23 February, talks were held between MAFF's Information Technology Directorate and senior vets on developing a database for recording information about FMD cases, including visits and restrictions. This system later became known as the Disease Control System. The principle behind it was the replacement of existing systems with a single, national database.

Building a new computer system, particularly one as large and complex as the Disease Control System, during a national crisis was exceptionally difficult. Months of work was compressed into two weeks. We commend the work of those involved in achieving this.

Geographical information systems

Accurate and up to date geographical information, including data on the limits of infected areas, the location and boundaries of infected premises and the spread and control of the disease, was vital to the effective management of the outbreak. MAFF set up a dedicated team at the Page Street Departmental Emergency Control Centre early on to handle the provision of this information.

MAFF's Geographical Information System was fed from two sources. The Disease Control System, which provided information on the addresses of infected premises and the Integrated Administration and Control System, or IACS, a business system used for payment of Common Agricultural Policy subsidies. IACS generated grid references for every field belonging to a particular farm, but it was not designed specifically for disease control purposes.

The main output of the Geographical Information System was a set of detailed maps made available centrally and to all the regions.

The Geographical Information System, and many of the decisions that were based on the data generated, particularly in relation to the 3km and contiguous culls, were the subject of often fierce criticism on the ground. As one farmer in Yorkshire told the Inquiry, *"what seems to be extraordinary is that there doesn't seem to be any link-up with all the work that the farmers have put in over the years doing their IACS registrations and all the field numbers and grid references"*.

Information was frequently out of date, on occasion by several years. It was sometimes difficult to pinpoint the location of livestock accommodation within an individual holding, or to identify the operator of the land.

There were particular difficulties with holdings covering more than one site. MAFF's recent attempts to rationalise the holding number system, gave rise to problems in identifying land ownership.

Many of the problems experienced by the Geographical Information System arose from the fact that one of the main elements had been designed for purposes other than that of controlling a major outbreak of a highly infectious animal disease. Many elements central to disease management, were not critical for payment of agricultural subsidies. Getting ahead of a disease as virulent as FMD permits little opportunity for challenging the data. It must be right first time.

If databases constructed for other purposes are to be used to support disease control they must be fit for that purpose in terms of design, accuracy and currency of data. However, it is preferable to design a system for the specific purpose of disease control.

19. **We recommend that DEFRA's Geographical Information System and the Integrated Administration and Control System (IACS) be designed so that they can be used more effectively for disease control purposes.**

Central data entry

The Government's Memorandum to this Inquiry (paragraph 2.8.14) stated that the Disease Control System "…was rolled out on 6 March 2001 and…was available both locally and to the Departmental Emergency Control Centre in Page Street". This was an overstatement.

On 6 March, the ability of regional Disease Control Centres to enter data on the system locally was limited. Information on how the outbreak was being handled on the ground had to be sent to Page Street from the regions by fax, phone or email and entered centrally.

However, by this stage, the regions were becoming increasingly beleaguered. Information gathering slipped down the list of priorities for the teams on the ground. As a result, the information fed into Page Street was patchy. To make matters worse, because of the relatively small number of staff at the centre, backlogs in data entry built up.

Central data entry was not going to be up to the task. Although MAFF again moved quickly to enable information to be entered locally, it was not until the end of April that the last local systems in the regions could be turned off. Even then, it took some effort to persuade certain Disease Control Centres to abandon the local systems in favour of one national system.

For at least three critical weeks in March, despite the effort that went into their development, systems for collecting key management information on the handling of the disease were ineffective. They remained only partially effective until the end of April 2001.

20. We recommend that DEFRA lay out milestones for investment and achievement for improved management information systems.

21. We recommend that data capture and management information systems be kept up to date and reflect best practice.

22. We recommend that the contingency plans of DEFRA, the Scottish Executive and the National Assembly for Wales specify the measures needed during an epidemic to monitor progress and report to key stakeholders.

23. We recommend that standard definitions of all important parameters of information be agreed in advance.

9.4 The tasks on the ground

On the ground, heroic efforts were made to tackle the infection and contain its spread.

In every area with significant presence of the virus a Disease Control Centre was established. The logistical effort involved was enormous, let alone the operational challenges facing the staff once the centres were set up. It is a tribute to everyone that so much was achieved in the face of the odds against them.

> "If you have a guy in a uniform who looks like he can go into the jungle and take people out; that's a really positive communication tool."

Senior Government Official
[of Brigadier Birtwhistle]

The outbreak was traumatic for everyone it touched. Many people sustained extreme working patterns, often 12 or more hours a day, seven days a week for long periods. They absorbed a great deal of emotion from farmers and others who were in considerable distress. Many staff, often at quite junior levels, endured abuse and intimidation.

Some suffered breakdowns. Some are still suffering.

Training on how to cope with stress was patchy. As the outbreak progressed, counselling and welfare provision was made increasingly available. However, it was not until April that some managers began to understand the need for staff to take a break from their duties.

Disease Control Centre staff were trained mainly on the job. At the start of the outbreak, there was a lack of clarity over roles. This was largely resolved by mid-April. However, it proved difficult in practice to disseminate lessons learned or best practice developed, because human resource management was focused principally on staff recruitment. Some good practice was developed, such as regular telephone conferences for Regional Operations Directors.

Regional Centres received many offers of help from the local community. However, there was no mechanism in place to manage this response, so many of them were unable to take up these offers. This gave rise to frustration and some resentment among local people.

24. **We recommend that contingency plans at regional level include mechanisms for making effective use of local voluntary resources.**

Efforts were focused, particularly in the early stages, on obtaining the large numbers of veterinary and administrative staff, and the goods and services necessary to mount an effective response to the disease.

Financial control systems were not up to the task. MAFF frequently had to pay over the odds in exchange for speed of delivery. The Department strayed from strict observance of its normal guidelines when awarding contracts.

The National Audit Office report contains a more detailed account of this aspect of the outbreak.

25. **We recommend that dedicated control systems be ready for use in a sustained emergency, and regularly tested as part of the contingency planning process.**

26. **We recommend that the processes for procuring and delivering the necessary goods and services from external sources during a crisis be reviewed. Systems should be tested to ensure they can cope with unexpected increased demands.**

27. **We recommend that priority be given to recruiting accounting and procurement professionals to operate in emergency control centres during a crisis.**

9.4.1 Setting up a Disease Control Centre

Setting up a Disease Control Centre was a complex operation. Considerable human, financial and material resources needed to be brought together very quickly.

For example, during the outbreak, the veterinary staff available to the Carlisle Centre increased from six to 200. Administrative staff rose from 31 to 250. At the peak there were 400 technical staff, compared to five before the outbreak. An entirely new force of 200 military personnel was brought in.

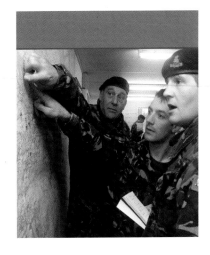

By the time the effort was at its peak, in April 2001, the Carlisle Disease Control Centre had acquired the following assets:

•	156	Portacabins & toilet blocks	•	720	Desks
•	217	Articulated wagons	•	838	Chairs
•	60	Eight-wheeler skip wagons	•	254	Cabinets
•	60	Eight-wheeler rigid wagons	•	316	Pedestals
•	8	Six-wheeler wagons	•	114	Fans
•	7	Four-wheeler wagons	•	67	Drawers
•	102	Telescopic handlers	•	31	Air conditioning units
•	22	Low loaders	•	16	Refrigerators
•	300	Hire cars	•	15	Book cases
•	6	Drinks machines	•	2	Boilers for coffee etc
•	8	Microwaves	•	62	Fax machines
•	5	Main servers	•	52	Server hubs
•	689	Computers	•	42	Photocopiers
•	114	Printers			

It was not just a question of getting hold of people and equipment, but also building the infrastructure. It needed telephone lines. It needed services such as electricity, water, gas and waste handling. Financial and personnel systems had to be put in place, including support mechanisms for staff many of whom were working under intense pressure. It needed effective channels of communication with the media and the local community. New staff needed basic training. The managers had to bring the whole thing together to make it work. Many staff were strangers to each other.

Setting up a Disease Control Centre represented a major achievement. Many people told us of their admiration and respect for the effort made by local staff. Nevertheless, the magnitude of the task reinforces several themes of our findings, including: the importance of thorough contingency planning involving everyone with an interest; the need for Government to mobilise its wider resources in a joined-up manner; the imperative for first-class communications with people in the local community affected by a crisis.

9.5 Slaughter policy and practice

Unprecedented numbers of animals were slaughtered during the outbreak, not only as a direct result of the disease control culling strategies but also because of the welfare problems caused by movement restrictions. The Livestock Welfare (Disposal) Scheme is discussed separately in section 12.7.

The basis of the control strategy was stamping out. This involved culling infected animals 'as soon as possible' coupled with the tracing and slaughtering of dangerous contacts, that is, animals thought to have been exposed to the disease. Other animals within a surveillance zone around the infected premises were then monitored closely. The Veterinary Instructions refer to 'slaughter with all practical speed' and 'immediate slaughter' following confirmation. There was perhaps an unstated assumption that confirmation itself would be speedy. In the early weeks, nothing was explicitly said to emphasise the importance of quick report-to-slaughter times. We discuss in section 10 the consequences of this.

Many of the circumstances during the 2001 epidemic were distressing for all concerned, including the farmers and their families whose animals were being destroyed, the vets supervising the destruction, the slaughtermen operating in conditions far removed from the automation of the abattoir. We heard harrowing accounts from many individuals during our regional visits. In some instances, many of which were reported in the media, slaughter was poorly carried out. The RSCPA expressed particular concern that piece rate payments to slaughtermen encouraged them to cut corners. The RSPCA received 130 complaints and investigated 83. While the aim must be to eliminate any cause for complaint, we believe these relatively low numbers show that in the majority of cases an unpleasant task was conducted effectively, often in very difficult conditions. Many farmers praised the manner in which the slaughtermen did their job. One submission said 'there were Government inadequacies in every area bar slaughter'.

But there were problems of delay. In the first few weeks of the outbreak, the ideal, only later made explicit, of slaughtering within 24 hours of report was very far from being met. In the first four weeks, one quarter to one third of infected premises were culled within 48 hours of owner report and only one in 10 was culled within 24 hours. Sometimes reports came in after dark: animals that were farmed extensively had to be gathered up; stockades had to be built; health and safety assessments had to be undertaken. Stock had to be valued and valuations were often disputed even though Veterinary Instructions limited the permissible delay to at most 12 hours.

The evidence presented to us did not confirm that valuation contributed significantly to delay. FMD status reports to the Joint Co-ordination Centre and COBR do not mention valuers as a problem whereas they do mention, for example, shortage of vets and slaughter equipment.

Nonetheless, it was suggested during March 2001 that valuation was causing delay. As a result, a system of standard values was introduced. Legislation did not allow compulsory standard values. The standard values were pitched generously to encourage farmers to take up the new system. In the event, only 4% of farmers made use of the standards. We heard evidence that the most significant effect of the standard valuation system was to inflate the value of culled animals, increasing the amount of compensation that had to be paid.

The standard valuation system was introduced to address a problem that may not have existed to any significant degree. It generated a new problem in its own right.

The valuation process and the financial implications for compensation are discussed in greater detail in the National Audit Office report. We return to compensation and insurance in section 17.

Before the introduction of slaughter on suspicion in late March there were delays of up to 96 hours while test results were awaited in around 12% of cases where diagnosis was uncertain.

Data supplied by DEFRA indicate that mean report-to-slaughter times were in the order of three days in the first weeks of the outbreak. The growing shortage of 'clean' veterinary resources limited the ability to maintain surveillance and tracing activity. In Cumbria, in an attempt to manage the scarcity of vets, a 'triage system' was introduced. This meant that, if a reported case with classic symptoms was within 3km of an existing case, then a less than fully-quarantined vet would be allowed to attend. On 10 March the Chief Veterinary Officer reduced the stand-down time for dirty vets from five to three days, stating that this was an 'informed' decision not simply a response to shortage of vets.

"I worked at one time or another with six slaughter teams. All were at least adequate and several of them were absolutely first class. …. Slaughter seemed to have processed very smoothly, and many owners commented on the smoothness and humanity of the operation."

Temporary Veterinary Inspector employed in Gloucester, 19 March – 19 April 2001

9.5.1 Slaughter and disposal of animals

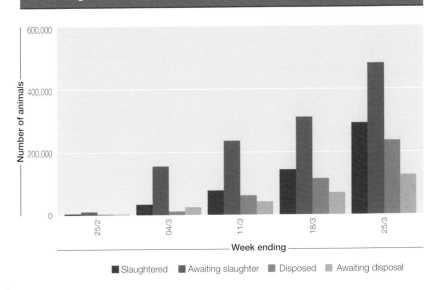

■ Slaughtered ■ Awaiting slaughter ■ Disposed ■ Awaiting disposal

Other parts of the Veterinary Instructions, relating to the presence of veterinary officers at slaughter, were compromised in some areas by scarce resources. The Royal College of Veterinary Surgeons submission to the Inquiry says that it was instrumental in reversing an attempt to reduce supervision of slaughter to as little as one Temporary Veterinary Inspector per 10 farms. A submission from a Temporary Veterinary Inspector made clear that the Royal College of Veterinary Surgeons accepted that some compromise of best practice was necessary given the other pressures of the outbreak. We also accept that there had to be some compromise given the unprecedented nature of events. But we believe that better contingency planning and speed of response could have limited the scale of the culling required and the associated need to compromise on good practice.

As the realisation grew that delays were occurring and contributing to spread, the pressure for further slaughter intensified. Slaughter on suspicion removed both the need to tie up a vet in surveillance of uncertain cases and the wait for test results. In mid May some 90% of slaughter on suspicion cases in sheep had been tested. Of these, between 5-10% tested positive. Slaughtering of stock on contiguous premises only occurred if the slaughter on suspicion case tested positive. The slaughter on suspicion policy put vets under pressure. We heard from many who were concerned at the number of animals culled on suspicion that subsequently tested negative.

Although relatively few submissions to the Inquiry raised the practicalities of the slaughter processes, some made proposals to enhance the efficiency and effectiveness of any future slaughter scenario. These include: conducting an audit of slaughter capacity, including those licensed to kill large animals, with a view to maintaining up-to-date records to draw on in an emergency; developing further a strategy for killing in the field where this proves necessary; considering an 'ID' or 'green card' system for licensed slaughterers; and banning the use of shotguns.

The RSPCA and the Humane Slaughter Association were present at some culls. A suggestion that slaughter should be open to independent observation by such organisations also warrants consideration provided that, in practice, this would not create additional potential for delay.

28. We recommend that DEFRA revise its guidance and instructions for slaughter.

9.7 Under control?

By Sunday 11 March, three weeks after the disease had broken out, 164 cases had been confirmed. A number of disease clusters had begun to emerge across the country (9.7.2). Disposal problems were mounting, particularly in Cumbria, where over 40,000 carcasses lay rotting on the ground. The rate of increase of animals awaiting slaughter was vastly outstripping the growing number of vets being deployed (9.7.1). The logistical machinery for dealing with the epidemic was inadequate for the task.

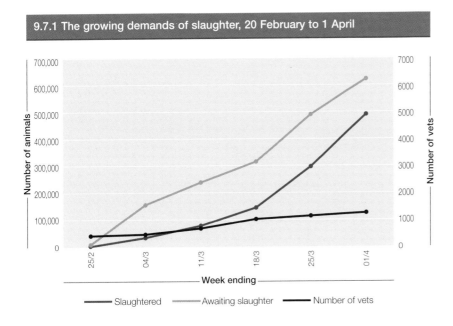

9.7.1 The growing demands of slaughter, 20 February to 1 April

Slaughtered — Awaiting slaughter — Number of vets

The process of tracing movements from Longtown market had been slow. MAFF had issued a news release the previous Thursday, 8 March, asking farmers for help in tracing sheep movements from Longtown as it believed that there was a substantial number of sales which took place 'out of the ring' by private transaction and which may not have been recorded. In an internal minute to officials on Friday 9 March, the Chief Veterinary Officer said it was difficult to ascertain the extent of the FMD outbreak and pointed to the following two weeks as being crucial in determining whether it would continue to escalate or level off.

On Sunday 11 March, the Minister of Agriculture, Nick Brown, during an interview on the BBC's Breakfast with Frost programme, made a number of comments to the effect that the disease was under control. Indeed he stressed that he was *absolutely certain*" that the disease was under control. A transcript of the interview is published in the CD-ROM annexes. The remarks were widely reported in the media on Monday 12 March and subsequently.

It is understandable that the Minister should have sought to reassure the public about control measures already in place. However, his comments did not reflect the situation on the ground. The disease was, at this stage, out of control by any reasonable measure (9.7.2). Thirty-four cases of FMD had

9.7.2 Map of the disease as at 0800 11 March 2001

○ Confirmed Cases

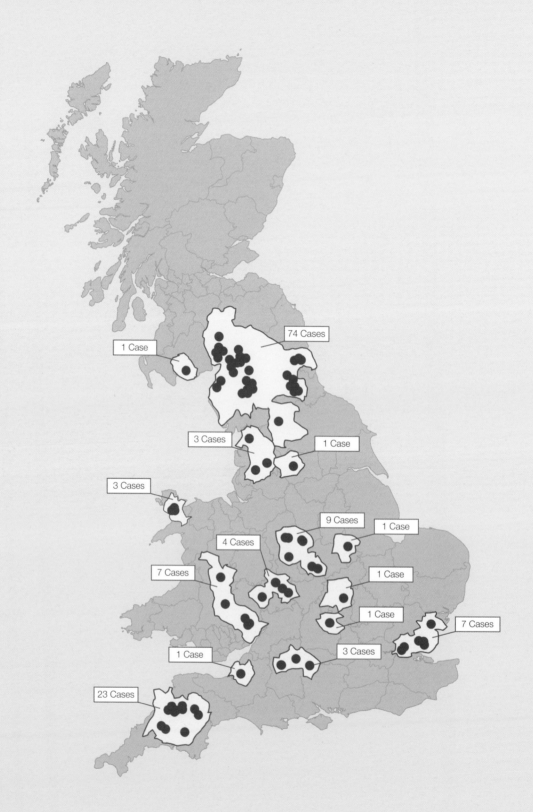

been confirmed in the two days leading up to the interview. A further 24 would be confirmed on 11 March. On 12 March, the day after the interview MAFF scientists, reporting internally the findings from their predictive computer models running in the previous week, made a tentative assessment that there might be 1,000-2,000 cases in total.

The Minister's comments contributed to the loss of trust on the part of rural communities. Many people, including some of those directly involved in managing the outbreak, still find it difficult to reconcile their experiences during this period with the notion of the disease being under control. The following extract comes from the transcript of one of the Inquiry's public meetings: *"…night after night on television news we had Jim Scudamore or Mr Brown, sometimes the Prime Minister, Professor King, it is under control, it is completely under control, it is definitely under control and we felt absolutely insulted and patronised by these lies that we were told. And furthermore it did a great deal of lasting damage because it meant that we are all now so completely cynical about anything the Government says. It has destroyed trust, trust takes years and years to build up and it can be destroyed overnight, and that is one thing that happened."*

The Minister's comments also sent a message to Government as a whole that the outbreak was being comprehensively managed by MAFF. It was another 11 days before COBR was opened (section 11).

9.8 The impact and timing of the involvement of the military

Of the many questions that were posed up and down the country at our public and round-table meetings, few were asked more often than: "Why, given the state of the disease, and the failure of the existing administrative structures to cope, were the armed forces not brought in sooner?" It is a compelling question to which there is no obvious answer.

We received many views. The delays may have been due to a desire to avoid sending negative political messages about the gravity of the crisis. They may have been caused by MAFF's reluctance to ask for help. Or they may have occurred simply because central government did not appreciate the sheer size of the task.

Whatever the reason, the arrival of the military heralded a positive step change in the management of the disease.

In fact, the Ministry of Defence had been alerted on 20 February to the possibility that the armed forces might be called upon to help. In response to a request from MAFF, the Ministry of Defence deployed a limited number of military vets on 14 March. By this time, however, the perception among the public and in the media was that the disease was running wild. Large numbers of decomposing carcasses were awaiting disposal, giving rise to both a general risk to public health and great distress for those directly affected. Calls for full-scale military deployment were growing.

Over the weekend of 17-18 March, two officers with expertise in logistics were despatched to MAFF headquarters to scope out the contribution the armed forces might make. Although the need to inform local military commanders to ensure that training manoeuvres did not aggravate the spread of the disease was set out clearly in the existing contingency plans, references to the role the armed forces might play in disease control were limited to the following: "If any emergency should arise where assistance from HM Forces is required, Head Office should be consulted immediately" – Veterinary Instructions chapter 3, paragraph 9.

The civilian authorities may have held the view that what the armed forces could best provide was large scale manpower to assist with slaughter, burial pits and disposal. In fact, that was not the case. There were ready sources of access to those. Brigadier Birtwhistle who eventually led the efforts to tackle the disease in Cumbria told the Inquiry, *"that is what the Yellow Pages is for"*. What was really lacking was logistical expertise and, more generally, the leadership and management skills needed to handle a crisis. As one farmer told the Inquiry, *"…one of the first things the army did when they moved in here was to find knowledgeable local people, they used local contractors, local hauliers and they used their knowledge to run their operation as efficiently as possible."*

The two officers' work over that weekend resulted in the deployment of military personnel in Devon on 19 March and Cumbria on 21 March, to be followed by further deployments in other regions. Critically, a Headquarters element of 101st Logistical Brigade was despatched to MAFF HQ on 23 March to assist with logistic co-ordination and planning. The Commander of the Brigade was subsequently appointed Deputy Director of Operations in the Joint Co-ordination Centre on 26 March.

The armed forces in the regions worked alongside the Regional Operations Directors and the existing Divisional Veterinary Managers. This approach was, in the worst affected areas, finally to bring the disease under control. This could and should have been done earlier.

However, we have been told by several senior officers that there may be circumstances under which the military is unable to provide support on the same scale as during this FMD outbreak. Military duties may mean that the availability of the armed forces to assist with the management of domestic crises is restricted.

29. **We recommend that as part of the mechanisms to trigger the wider Government response, the military be consulted at the earliest appropriate opportunity to provide advice and consider the nature of possible support.**

30. **We recommend that as part of its contingency planning, DEFRA, the Scottish Executive and the National Assembly for Wales, working with the Civil Contingencies Secretariat, examine the practicality of establishing a national volunteer reserve trained and informed to respond immediately to an outbreak of infectious animal disease.**

9.9 Scotland

In Scotland, action was more rapid. The first outbreak was confirmed in Lockerbie on 1 March. Immediately, an operation swung into action to manage the emergency. This was, in our view, an example of the disease outbreak being handled as effectively as possible given the circumstances. Without doubt, the experience of the Lockerbie air disaster some 12 years earlier facilitated cross-agency working. This was not, however, the critical factor. Other areas of Britain without such experiences were effective – Staffordshire and Lancashire being good examples. The components of the effective response shown in Scotland were as follows: proper planning and rehearsals; access to all the senior people in the relevant agencies; short chains of command up to and down from the centre; decision making devolved as far as possible to local level; good management information systems; effective computer systems and links; effective communications internally, and externally both with the media and with key stakeholders.

In section 10, we set out the role that the Scottish Executive played in the development of the 3km sheep cull north of the border. Some people have argued that, given the devolution on policy on animal health matters to Scotland, there should also be devolution of the role of the State Veterinary Service. On the face of it, it is an unusual arrangement whereby policy on animal health is devolved to Edinburgh, whereas field operations work is still governed from London. However, infectious diseases do not recognise internal boundaries and borders. We believe therefore that the existing arrangements and a national State Veterinary Service should be maintained and do not recommend any further devolution of the Service in Scotland. Sensible local delegated responsibilities are already in place and worked well during the 2001 epidemic.

9.10 Wales

The National Assembly for Wales has published its own assessment of the outbreak and lessons to be learned (in the CD-ROM annexes). The National Audit Office's summary has also been reproduced, in the appendices to the Inquiry Report. In contrast to Scotland, the National Assembly for Wales lacked full legal powers to take decisions alone on disease control. It was able to make legislation separately on imports and exports but had no role to play in the declaratory orders designating infected areas in Wales. It had no power to make decisions on animal movement restrictions. In accordance with the Animal Health Act 1981 and the Transfer of Functions Order 1999 (SI999/672), the National Assembly for Wales legislated jointly with the Department, nationally, to enable a consistent and uniform approach to be undertaken by the enforcement bodies.

> "When agriculture suffers disease or other shocks the knock on effect to the rest of the rural economy is sharp and severe."
>
> *Country Land and Business Association*

This was a significant source of tension. The then Minister of Rural Affairs, Carwyn Jones, told us that he was seen as politically responsible for the management of the crisis in Wales even though, constitutionally, he was not. He had held daily press conferences for the first month and regularly thereafter. The National Assembly for Wales had also set up telephone helplines about the outbreak. The fact that information was being imparted in this way reinforced assumptions that the National Assembly for Wales was taking decisions and had legal powers to act alone.

The National Assembly for Wales has identified several occasions, particularly with regards to changes to the licensed movement regime, when it failed to find out about significant policy decisions or developments until the last moment, leaving little time to prepare staff on the ground or brief Assembly Ministers. Despite the presence of Assembly staff in London acting as a link with departments in London and COBR, the pace of developments meant that communications were sometimes confused. The Minister told us that he needed the same legal powers as his Scottish counterpart, although this was not a call for a separate State Veterinary Service.

Political responsibility without power is uncomfortable. We understand why the National Assembly for Wales believes that it should be given constitutional powers, and the appropriate resources for animal health issues related to disease control in Wales. We are not convinced, however, that further fragmenting disease control policy is the best way forward. As we have said in relation to Scotland, exotic animal diseases, such as FMD, do not respect borders and so there is a strong argument in favour of retaining a uniform policy of disease control in England and Wales, which can be directed from the centre but adapted to local circumstances. The relationship between the National Assembly for Wales and DEFRA needs to revisited, however, in the context of contingency planning for future outbreaks to ensure that there are clear lines of responsibility, accountability and communication.

31. **We recommend that the National Assembly for Wales and DEFRA develop a comprehensive agreement for co-ordinating the management of outbreaks of infectious animal diseases in Wales. This should cover all aspects of a disease outbreak, delegating responsibility locally, where appropriate, and providing clear lines of communication and accountability.**

9.11 Wider rural impact and its costs

Alongside developments in disease control there was a growing recognition of the wider impact that the disease and the control measures were having. In particular, the closure of footpaths was having a considerable impact on tourism and the wider rural economy. *"About two weeks in to the outbreak, the closure of footpaths outside the Infected Areas had provoked regional colleagues to contact the Department of Environment, Transport and the Regions expressing worries about the potential impact of this policy. At this stage, there had still been the expectation that the outbreak would be over by the early summer so discussion with concerned parties such as the National Trust had focused on how to encourage visitors to return once the outbreak was over."* Senior Official, Department of Environment, Transport and the Regions.

Farming and tourism are interdependent and interlinked with the wider rural economy. Rural tourism and other businesses are often dependent on access to a landscape heavily influenced by farming. Many rural areas have a narrow economic base, dominated by farming and tourism; and many rural businesses are vulnerable, for example where they depend on passing trade.

In addition to the direct impact on hotels, holiday lettings and visitor attractions, other examples of rural activity were affected by FMD control measures. Village services such as pubs, shops and post offices; voluntary organisations dependent on countryside recreation, leisure activities and outdoor sporting events all suffered.

Section 14 discusses estimates of the overall economic costs of the outbreak.

Some of the hardest hit regions have below average incomes. Devon and Cumbria were hit particularly hard, both because of the extent of the outbreak and the relative importance of tourism compared to livestock in these regions. Tourism contributes 6% to the GDP of both Cumbria and Devon compared to agriculture, arable and livestock, which contributes 4%.

In early April 2001, the Department of Environment, Transport and the Regions asked the Government Offices in England to commission surveys to assess the economic impact in their regions. Some impact assessment work was also done by the Department for Culture, Media and Sport, based on tourism surveys. Over 40% of businesses in Cumbria, Devon and Cornwall surveyed in April/May 2001 reported that they had been adversely affected, compared to just over 30% in the South West and North West as a whole. The GDP loss to the whole of the South West in March and April was estimated at just over 3%, while lost turnover was around £760m.

The Rural Task Force

As the disease spread, an appreciation grew of the wider implications for the rural economy. In response, the Government established the Rural Task Force which met first on 14 March. The Rural Task Force included representatives of a range of Government departments and agencies, and of stakeholders from farming, tourism, local government, small business, conservation and community interests. Its remit was to consider the consequences of FMD for the rural economy, both immediately and in the longer term, and to report to the Prime Minister on appropriate measures.

The final report of the Rural Task Force 'Tackling the Impact of Foot and Mouth Disease on the Rural Economy' was published on 18 October.

Throughout our Inquiry many people have commented that the Rural Task Force played a significant role in increasing wider awareness of the impact of FMD beyond just the farming community. In particular the Rural Task Force played an important role in introducing a risk based approach to the re-opening of footpaths and tourist attractions closed as a result of the disease.

Both the Department of Environment, Transport and the Regions and stakeholders welcomed the Rural Task Force forum and felt that it had made a valuable contribution. However, it was not seen as the whole answer. *"There should have been some mechanism to enable a wider consideration of the policy issues. Discussion of policy issues elsewhere had usually been firmly focused on fighting a war against FMD, without full consideration of the potential impact on the rural economy."* *Senior Official, Department of Environment, Transport and the Regions.*

32. **We recommend that, where the control of exotic animal diseases has wider economic or other implications, the Government ensure that those consequences for the country as a whole are fully considered.**

9.12 The Regional Operations Director system strengthened

As the disease progressed, it became increasingly clear that the policy of placing overall responsibility for regional management of the disease in the hands of the local Divisional Veterinary Manager was not working. This was not due to any inherent lack of capability on the part of the individuals concerned. Rather, the failure to cope with an outbreak of this scale meant that it was important to avoid wasting vital veterinary resources on work that could be done by other, non-specialist, staff or contractors. Remedying this situation became pressing.

The desirability of identifying an individual to manage regional stakeholders and external relationships was recognised by MAFF senior management early on. Given the need to release veterinary resources, this role developed to encompass the management of all non-veterinary work in the regions, including administration and media relations.

The first Regional Operations Directors, both MAFF senior civil servants, were appointed to head the Disease Control Centres in Cumbria and Devon on 19 March. Further appointments were made to a number of other Disease Control Centres over the following days. The introduction of the Regional Operations Directors made a big contribution to the fight against the disease.

Relationships within the Disease Control Centre were often tense. There were multiple lines of control, with administrative, veterinary and military elements. Finding a way through and managing these tensions successfully, depended very heavily on the personal abilities of senior management, particularly the Regional Operations Directors.

Regional Operations Directors often held their posts for relatively short periods. For example, the first director at the Carlisle Disease Control Centre remained in post for just six weeks. We commend this practice, on the basis that the demands of the job were such that individuals needed to be rested in order to remain effective.

Preparations should be made, through the contingency planning process, to appoint Regional Operations Directors very much earlier, ideally as soon as an outbreak is identified. The Permanent Secretary of DEFRA told the Inquiry that, in future, Regional Operations Directors would be employed immediately.

33. **We recommend that contingency plans provide for early appointment of Regional Operations Directors or their equivalent to take on operational management of a crisis. There should be a cadre of senior managers – not all of whom need come from central government – who can fulfil the role of the Regional Operations Director in an emergency and who should be trained in advance.**

In addition, although Regional Operations Directors made a positive contribution in every case, their effectiveness depended on the individual calibre of those appointed. As the Permanent Secretary of DEFRA, put it, *"outstanding individuals could achieve outstanding results"*. We believe that proper training and sharing of expertise would allow individual calibre, and hence effectiveness, to flourish. This should include training in communication with the media and local communities. The role of the Regional Operations Director is focused very tightly on local delivery. He or she represents the sharp end of the Government response in the regions.

10.1 Background

Around 10 March, the Chief Veterinary Officer was realising that the existing policies of infected premises slaughter together with tracing and slaughter of dangerous contacts, were not containing the epidemic. Information available at the time could not fully explain why this was so. Either the policies themselves were inadequate or they were not being fully implemented or, to some degree, both.

The number of infected premises was doubling every week. The epidemic was on track to overwhelm resources. Around the country, including at MAFF's Page Street Headquarters, the notion was growing that new instruments of policy were needed. MAFF's Veterinary Management meetings pondered options for increasing the culling of sheep. Pre-emptive slaughter of sheep on Dartmoor was considered, focusing on premises contiguous to infected animals, as was a cull of all fat-stock sheep. The Chief Veterinary Officer was also considering extending the definition of 'dangerous contact'.

The epidemiologists at the Veterinary Laboratories Agency were simulating the epidemic on computers using the InterSpread model. By 12 March, they were forecasting that it might reach between 1,000 and 2,000 cases, compared with the 182 so far confirmed.

In Scotland, the Scottish Executive, working very closely with the NFU Scotland, had started to contemplate unprecedented steps in an effort to control an increasingly desperate situation. The epidemic in Dumfries and Galloway was exploding, threatening the valuable cattle populations to the north. Informally at first and, as far as we have been able to discover, without any scientific advice, plans were rapidly worked out for a 3km pre-emptive sheep cull. All sheep within 3km of a confirmed infected premises would be slaughtered. Meetings with MAFF in London and at Downing Street were called urgently and agreement quickly reached to coordinate policy across the Scottish-English border.

On 15 March, these policies were announced simultaneously in Scotland and England, although they were not implemented until 22 and 28 March respectively. The fact that the Minister of Agriculture, Nick Brown, announced that "animals within the 3km zones" were to be destroyed on a precautionary basis, without explicitly excluding cattle, caused confusion and consternation. Although a clarification was made later in the day that cattle were specifically excluded from this policy, resentment remained and affected local attitudes. The scene was set for confrontation.

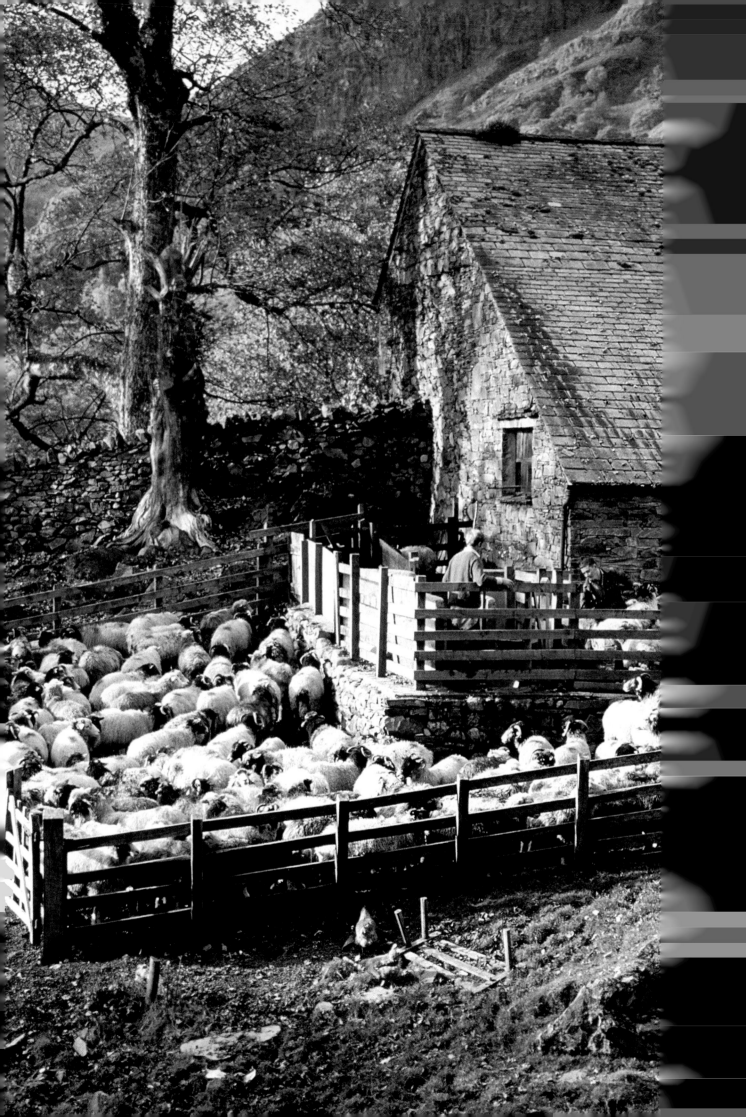

10.2 The genesis of the FMD Science Group

If we step back from these events and return to late February, in parallel with the activity of the State Veterinary Service and MAFF, Sir John Krebs, Chairman of the Food Standards Agency was concerned how the FMD outbreak might develop. Before the end of the month, he was already speaking to a number of experts in epidemiological modelling to seek their views. Following these discussions an ad hoc group was hosted by the Food Standards Agency on 6 March. The epidemiologists discussed their initial view of the outbreak and what information they needed from MAFF to help analyse and predict the progress of the emerging epidemic. MAFF supplied the data requested on 13 March. Four groups of epidemiologists began their analysis. The Imperial College team (some of whom had recently published an analysis of FMD data from the 1967/8 outbreak) was the most advanced at this stage. On 16 March they sent MAFF their initial view that the critical challenge was to reduce the delay between report and slaughter. They also hoped that the 3km cull announced the day before would, when implemented, improve matters.

The epidemiologists met again on 21 March at the Food Standards Agency. Professor David King, the Government's Chief Scientific Adviser, and the Chief Veterinary Officer were among those present. The conclusions of all the forecasts were bleak. The models had been constructed independently,

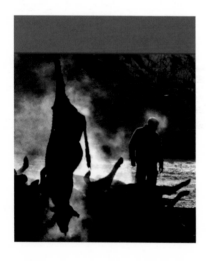

10.2.1 "Out of control" – the R_0 number

The epidemiologists had looked at what was happening to the so called 'case reproduction number', R_0 which is the average number of new cases generated by one current case.

Suppose there are FMD cases on 10 farms. How many new farms will these infect? With no movement restrictions or any kind of culling, it might be 50, corresponding to an R_0 value of 5. With movement restrictions and culling of infected herds it might be 15, an R_0 value of 1.5. These newly infected farms will go on to infect further farms. As long as R_0 is greater than one, then the number of new cases at each stage continues to increase and the epidemic is out of control. To get the epidemic under control, R_0 has to be reduced below one, so that the 10 current cases directly cause fewer than 10 new cases. To be sure of stopping the epidemic quickly, getting R_0 to a smaller value, say 0.5, is a good idea if possible. But keeping R_0 below 1 is the prime aim of any policy for managing an epidemic.

Preliminary data from the 2001 UK FMD epidemic implied that, early in the outbreak, on average, one infected premise had infected 1.2 other farms by 24 hours after its own infection was discovered. Thus, even a perfectly implemented cull of infected premises within 24 hours of discovery would not, on its own, have controlled that epidemic until the disease itself had reduced the density of susceptible farms to such an extent that the epidemic ended naturally.

10.2.2 The role of the FMD Science Group in informing policy

The analytical evidence presented by the Science Group was seized upon by decision-makers in a situation where hard evidence was difficult to come by. The policy decisions that were underpinned by the Group's analysis were contentious. Yet the creation, constitution and operation of the Science Group did not conform completely with the Office of Science and Technology's guidelines on scientific advice and policy making, nor take cognisance of the lessons drawn by The BSE Inquiry[3]. The genesis of the Group was a decision to bring together a particular group of experts – epidemiological modellers – to inform the Food Standards Agency. Although other scientific disciplines were represented this led some people to comment that the group was more of a 'modelling sub-committee' than a full FMD Science Group. That the group was open to such criticism was unhelpful.

The Science Group epidemiologists are world experts in their field. Many of the public accusations levelled at their work are based on limited knowledge of the statistical and mathematical techniques they employed, for example to address weaknesses in the raw data. Nonetheless, the highly specialist nature of their work made it difficult for other FMD experts to engage with the detail, especially when they themselves were under huge pressure of work in managing the outbreak. At times there were polarised views within the group but no convincing mechanism for handling conflicts of opinion.

The membership of the Group was gradually extended, with increased veterinary input. By this stage the contentious decisions had already been taken.

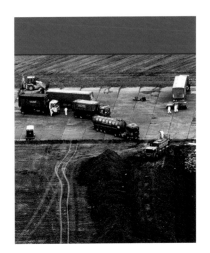

each on different principles, but their fundamental conclusion was the same. The disease was out of control (10.2.1).

These matters were now seen to have much wider implications for the whole of government. So, from then on, the Chief Scientific Adviser took the lead. Building on the group that met at the Food Standards Agency he created the FMD Science Group which met regularly from 26 March until 1 November (31 meetings in all).

34. We recommend that DEFRA's Chief Scientist maintain a properly constituted standing committee ready to advise in an emergency on scientific aspects of disease control. The role of this group should include advising on horizon scanning and emerging risks. Particular attention should be given to the recommendations on the use of scientific advisory committees in The BSE Inquiry report of 2000.

3 The BSE Inquiry: the Inquiry into BSE and variant CJD in the United Kingdom, 2000.

"…it was the right decision to take, the contiguous cull, and if the contiguous cull was done at Willy Cleave's farm when his sheep were all in the shed and the surrounding farms were all contiguously culled out that would have been the end of foot and mouth in Devon."

Public Meeting,
regional visit to the South West

10.3 The emergence of the contiguous cull

By 21 March, the Chief Veterinary Officer and the epidemiologists in the State Veterinary Service, along with those of the Chief Scientific Adviser and groups of independent epidemiological modellers were all coming to the same conclusion. Existing policies were not yet controlling the spread of the disease. Something needed to be done and done fast.

The findings of the 21 March modelling meeting were due to be sent to MAFF so that it could make a policy announcement later in the week. However, although there had been agreement at the 21 March meeting "that individuals would not talk to the media", Professor Roy Anderson, Head of Infectious Disease Epidemiology at Imperial College, stuck to a pre-arranged appearance on the BBC's 'Newsnight' that evening. He did not discuss the details of that afternoon's meeting but he did say *"I think everybody is in agreement, both government, the farming community and the independent scientific advice, that this epidemic is not under control at the current point in time"*. He went on to say *"If this cull [i.e. the 3km cull in Cumbria, Dumfries and Galloway announced on 15 March] is applied vigorously and effectively enough you could turn the epidemic in to a decaying process hopefully within, a month to two months. Doing something even better than that I am not convinced is possible at the moment."*

Professor Anderson's intervention on 21 March forced the pace of developments, bringing into public discussion the notion that the outbreak was out of control.

On 23 March, at a press conference with the Minister of Agriculture, Nick Brown, Professor King reiterated that the epidemic was out of control. Subsequent press reports on 24 March said that the time between report and slaughter needed to be brought down to 24 hours. Some suggested that the recently announced 3km sheep cull, which had only begun to be implemented in Scotland two days previously and would not be started in Cumbria for another four days, would need to be extended. Others alluded to a 1.5km ring cull of all susceptible animals.

We have been unable to find a clear account of decision making around that time. The pressure on the Government from all sides was growing. The press reports on 24 March talked of 'confusion'. Some suggested that the Prime Minister had already given the order for a pre-emptive cull. Tensions were rising. The MAFF Permanent Secretary, Brian Bender, told us that, between 21 and 26 March, there was a great deal of confusion. The epidemiological modellers were concentrating on the principal factors influencing the spread of disease from an infected place to neighbouring farms. The vets, desperately short of resources and knowing that they were failing to deliver the critically important rapid slaughter of infected animals, were also considering extending the definition of dangerous contacts to bring more animals into the culling net. Everyone involved accepted that the slaughter of infected cases as rapidly as possible and certainly within 24 hours of report or less was the priority but that this, on its own, would not be enough to contain the disease at this stage. Some believed that enhanced biosecurity was what was needed, but the resources were not available to realise fully the biosecurity measures already in place.

It has become apparent to us that, while some policy decisions were recorded with commendable clarity, some of the most important ones taken during the outbreak were recorded in the most perfunctory way, and sometimes not at all. In the context of our own Inquiry, this has made the task of constructing an audit trail extremely difficult in some vital policy areas, including the contiguous and 3km culls, and the decision to close footpaths.

Good record keeping is essential. Records are not kept purely to inform potential future Inquiries. They should set out what has to be done, when and by whom, to help ensure that results are delivered.

35. We recommend that, from day one of an outbreak, provision be made to keep a record of all decisions made and any actions to be taken.

The Chief Veterinary Officer feared that a national 3km pre-emptive cull was neither practical nor likely to be legal (17.3). Professor King told us that, in the period between 21 and 24 March, he had asked the Imperial College team to model smaller radii than 3km. On the basis of that modelling, a radius of between 1 and 1.5km had appeared to be optimum in bringing the epidemic under control with the minimum necessary cull. Somewhere in the midst of this the idea was born that a contiguous premises cull would have a similar impact to a 1.5km cull, although the FMD Science Group was to be asked to advise on the definition of 'contiguous' during the following weeks.

The models showed that a national policy based on slaughter of infected animals within 24 hours of report and the pre-emptive slaughter of all animals on contiguous premises would contain the disease and eventually eliminate it while minimising the total number of animals slaughtered, compared with the other scenarios that had been modelled (10.3.1). This led to the introduction of the so-called 24/48 hours slaughter policy.

We have been unable to establish the precise rationale for the target of 48 hours, nor ascertain the source of that timescale. Professor King told us that it was designed to allow for the prioritisation of infected premises culling and that it recognised that the incubation period gave some time for manoeuvre in tackling contiguous premises. The target of 48 hours was first stated in the Number 10 lobby briefing on the morning of 26 March. It formed part of the Minister's statement to the House of Commons, which formally confirmed the new policy, on 27 March. We have been unable to establish any formal record of the decision to introduce the 48 hour target. For what became such a central component of disease control policy, albeit one that proved unattainable in practice, this is regrettable.

10.3.1 Predicted impact of culling policies

Chart A

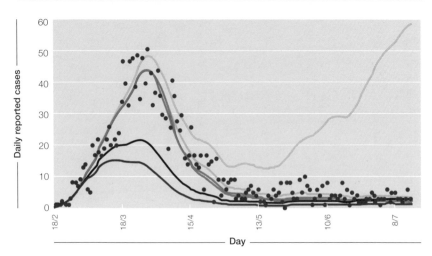

• Numbers of cases

Scenarios

(1) Actual epidemic – culling as occurred (1848 cases by 16 July & 7650 farms culled)

(2) 24h IP from April, non-IP culling as occurred (10% case decrease, 8% cull decrease)

(3) IP as occurred, 48h CP culling from April (9% case decrease, 24% cull decrease)

(4) 24h IP from start, non-IP culling as occurred (47% case decrease, 42% cull decrease)

(5) 24h IP, 48h CP culling from start (66% case decrease, 62% cull decrease)

(6) IP culling as occurred, no non-IP culling (114% case increase, 50% cull decrease)

Chart B

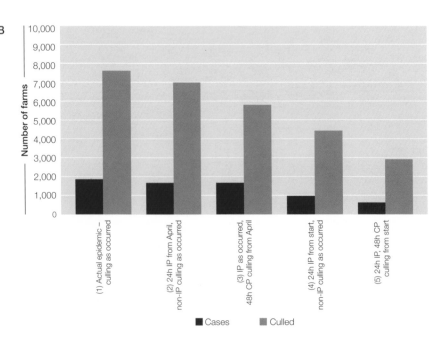

Source: Ferguson et al.[4] (Data at 16 July 2001)

The epidemiologists modelled different scenarios. These include various culling policies:

• culling infected premises (IP or FMD cases) within 24 hours of report
• pre-emptive culling of non-infected premises (non-IP), namely dangerous contacts and contiguous premises (CP)
• contiguous premises culling within 48 hours.

Implementation of all these policies was modelled:

• from the start of the outbreak
• from 1 April 2001.

What actually happened in practice was also represented on the computer, for comparison.

10.3.1 Predicted impact of culling policies – additional notes continued

Each scenario has a different impact on the shape of the epidemic (chart A) and on the numbers of FMD cases and farms culled out in total (chart B). What happened in the actual epidemic (scenario 1) can be compared with the theoretical scenarios. The models were calculated using farm numbers, rather than numbers of animals, at July 2001. Farms culled for welfare reasons were not included.

Timing of the slaughter of infected premises has the most significant effect on the size of the epidemic. Had the 24 hour target for infected premises been achieved from the start, the epidemic would have been dramatically reduced. (Compare scenarios 1 and 5 in chart B.)

However, culling of infected premises alone would not have eradicated the disease. The modelling suggests that, without any non-infected premises culling, the epidemic would have been catastrophic (scenario 6 in chart A). Not only does the culling of non-infected premises reduce the predicted number of FMD cases, but it also – perhaps counter-intuitively – reduces the total number of farms culled (for example, compare scenarios 4 and 5 in chart B). Thus, overall, appropriate pre-emptive culling reduces the numbers affected by the epidemic and its duration.

[4] Transmission intensity and impact of control policies on the foot and mouth epidemic in Great Britain. Ferguson et al. Nature (2001) 413, 542-548

10.4 Slaughter on suspicion

In practice, the 48 hour contiguous cull was probably never more than 50% implemented. Certainly, in the areas of the highest infectivity, the implementation rate was lowest. But efforts to slaughter infected premises within 24 hours of report (rather than confirmation) increased dramatically along with monitoring of success. Before 22 March, when a vet felt unable to confirm a case on clinical grounds but was equally unable to be sure there was no infection, samples were taken and tests carried out. Only if these proved positive were the animals slaughtered. This testing could take up to four days so infected animals could be left alive for up to five days. Slaughter on suspicion was introduced on 24 March, requiring slaughter of all suspicious animals whether clinically confirmed or not.

This policy highlighted the tension between the need for speed and the desire for certainty of diagnosis. In the event only a small proportion of sheep slaughtered on suspicion subsequently tested positive. This led people to call for the use of rapid on-farm tests and technologies which were being newly developed (10.4.1). These technologies drew upon standard laboratory techniques and some people argued that, as they were available, they should be used. However the tests they could perform in the field had not been validated to the same standards as conventional laboratory tests. It would have been inappropriate to use potentially unreliable tests during the FMD crisis.

Rapid diagnostic tools could be of considerable value by supporting clinical judgement and, potentially, improving the quality of decision making on the ground. For the last few years, the Pirbright Laboratory has been developing pen-side tests for detecting FMD virus. These are test sticks, based on the technology used in home pregnancy tests, and give rapid results within a few minutes. Limited but encouraging trials have been conducted in the field to date.

36. **We recommend that the State Veterinary Service be routinely equipped with the most up-to-date diagnostic tools for use in clinical practice, to contribute to speed and certainty of action at critical times.**

"One of the major lessons of the 1997 (classical swine fever) outbreak (in The Netherlands) was that the suspension of the preventative killing of suspected holdings resulted in massive spread of infection. This was subsequently identified as a major mistake in the reviews of that outbreak. Clearly this was a factor in the policy approach followed [in 2001] by our Dutch colleagues."

Commissioner David Byrne, response to the European Parliament Temporary Committee on FMD, 25 March 2002

10.4.1 Developing rapid on-farm tests

One specific offer of testing came from the Agricultural Research Service of the United States Department of Agriculture. In collaboration with private companies, the Agricultural Research Service had developed a Real-Time Polymerase Chain Reaction (RT-PCR) test using portable equipment, such as the 'SmartCycler'. US scientists offered to visit the Pirbright Laboratory with their equipment and materials in order to test them under field conditions during the UK outbreak but the priorities of managing the outbreak made this impracticable.

The Agricultural Research Service claimed that their tests which give results in a couple of hours were straightforward and reliable. However, they wished to publish their results in the scientific journals before proceeding to validation.

The Pirbright Laboratory and the FMD Science Group considered the technology carefully. Pirbright Laboratory uses RT-PCR routinely in the laboratory and had evaluated the use of portable equipment. They concluded that RT-PCR has much potential for rapid testing in mobile or local laboratories, but not on the farm itself.

RT-PCR goes through cycles of copying specific sequences of DNA which, if present, can then be visualised. It is a sensitive technique which allows pre-clinical detection of small amounts of FMD virus within a couple of hours. Contamination can lead to false positives. In the field RT-PCR can be unreliable, resulting in false negatives.

10.5 The justification of the contiguous cull

The justification for culling contiguous premises was founded on a statistical concept. All the models showed that culling farms neighbouring infected premises would reduce spread of infection and control the epidemic. This was based on the observation that, on average, animals on 34% of premises within a radius of 1.5km of infected premises came down with FMD. Although culling contiguous premises was a blunt policy instrument, it had the benefit of speed in decision making. It did not depend on the epidemiological groundwork to identify dangerous contacts, which was resource intensive and time consuming.

From some perspectives the rigorous application of a contiguous culling policy was a desperate measure. But the situation was desperate. The epidemic was expanding out of control. FMD could have become endemic. The pressure was intense. Resources were stretched. There was no time to explore alternatives or carry out experiments. Here was a simple formula that both the Chief Veterinary Officer and the Chief Scientific Adviser said would work. And that was the advice that was followed.

10.6 Implementing the culling policies

MAFF now had a range of culling policies to be implemented on the ground:

- Culling of all susceptible animals on premises with clinically confirmed cases within 24 hours of report.
- Slaughter on suspicion.
- Culling of known dangerous contacts.
- Culling of sheep, pigs and goats within 3km of infected premises in Cumbria and Dumfries and Galloway.
- Culling of all susceptible animals contiguous to infected premises within 48 hours.

Vets in MAFF Headquarters at Page Street and around the regions had to organise all this and communicate the details to everyone concerned. There was little time for reflection or any opportunity to think through all the issues. And many complex issues were to arise.

The 3km cull was controversial in Cumbria though less so in Scotland. The contiguous cull was controversial wherever it was rigorously applied. Many representations were made to us by farmers. They believed they were victims of the unthinking application of a generic policy in spite of obvious local circumstances and mitigating factors that should have been considered. In Scotland the contiguous cull policy was not generally applied. It was instead used strategically to help control spread at the edge of the epidemic.

Many farmers did not understand or accept the statistical basis for the policy. Most contiguous premises were not infected and probably would not have become infected. But some would and, if not culled out, would have revealed themselves only when they had contributed to the further spread of disease.

Many vets accepted this and had no professional doubts. But some, including many Temporary Veterinary Inspectors, did not. They called for more local discretion. However, introducing widespread discretion was judged not to be wise at the height of the epidemic.

There were numerous appeals against the contiguous cull and many of these were upheld. In several instances the farm in question was re-designated as not contiguous. A climate of confrontation and opposition to the cull was generated in many parts of the country.

The experience in Scotland at this stage is illuminating. Through the State Veterinary Service, the Scots were implementing national policies but, because of the powers vested in the Scottish Minister, there was considerable local discretion. First, with the help of the NFU Scotland, it had been possible to explain the rationale and to build a reasonable consensus in support of the 3km sheep cull in Dumfries and Galloway. In other words, communication of the policy goals was successful. Second, a decision was taken to apply the contiguous culling policy pragmatically and only in those premises at the edge of the epidemic zone as an extra precaution to prevent the spread of infection into new territory. These policies worked well. The disease was eliminated after 91 days.

"The contiguous cull was the single most controversial policy initiative of the entire battle against Foot and Mouth disease. It was crude, medieval and extremely brutal. And the fact that it was stepped up when the General Election loomed closer made many suspicious that it was driven by politics, not science."

Editorial, Western Morning News, 22/05/02

10.6.1 Anglesey

The dense cluster of infection on the Isle of Anglesey made it feasible to implement a more radical culling policy from late March to mid April. This involved removing all sheep in a geographically defined area.

The policy was effective in stamping out the virus on Anglesey but led to a higher number of animals being culled per infected premises than in the rest of Wales. Thus, 4,235 animals were culled per infected premises whereas elsewhere in Wales the average was 2,779. The then Welsh Minister of Rural Affairs, Carwyn Jones, suggested to the Inquiry that the cull was widely supported by local farmers as the approach was simple and equitable. Nevertheless a small group of farmers mounted a legal challenge and were able to keep their animals.

The Anglesey cull was an example of how policy could be tailored to local circumstances. Elsewhere in Wales the pattern of disease was less dense and culling on the Anglesey model was not a viable option.

In an FMD outbreak tight central direction is necessary both at the early stages of the epidemic and as it reaches its height. Good epidemiological judgements are only possible when all relevant factors are taken into account. This is one reason why reference had to be made to the State Veterinary Service specialists in Page Street. When eventually the Chief Veterinary Officer saw the epidemic was tailing off, more local discretion became possible. From 26 April the rules governing the contiguous cull were altered.

37. **We recommend that in order to build support steps always be taken to explain the rationale of policies on the ground, particularly where implementation is likely to be controversial. Wherever possible, local circumstances should be taken into account without undermining the overall strategy.**

The introduction of the explicit 24 hour report to slaughter policy (including slaughter on suspicion) and the contiguous cull policy played a critical part in disease control in the 2001 outbreak. The Government felt it had little choice but to accept the advice it received on these matters from the Chief Veterinary Officer and the Chief Scientific Adviser. But the process of determining and responding to that advice should have been better. It was certainly not in line with the recommendations on scientific advice made by The BSE Inquiry. Communication of the rationale generally was poor. The decision making process remains unclear. In some cases too the statutory position was insufficiently clear. Although the circumstances which led to this were exceptional, it was in part a failure of advance planning.

The possibility of adopting a contiguous culling policy in future should be retained. However, it is imperative that it should only be applied in the light of up-to-date scientific and veterinary advice. Robust management information should be available to support any decision.

The rationale must be discussed with stakeholders and understood in advance by those who may be affected, as part of the strategic preparations for disease control. This position supports the general conclusion that draconian steps at the beginning of an outbreak are likely to produce a favourable end result in terms of cost and numbers of animals slaughtered. A more discretionary approach may be introduced once the picture becomes clearer.

There are many lessons here for contingency planning, for clear communication of policy rationale to those most affected and for a wider understanding of the circumstances where local discretion may be applied.

38. **We recommend that provision be made for the possible application of pre-emptive culling policies, if justified by well-informed veterinary and scientific advice, and judged to be appropriate to the circumstances.**

11.1 Opening of COBR

By the morning of Thursday 22 March the situation was dire. The number of new cases over the previous week had averaged 31 each day. Following an emergency morning meeting with the Prime Minister, the Minister for Agriculture and others at Number 10 to discuss options for tackling the rapidly escalating crisis, the Cabinet Secretary gave instructions for the Cabinet Office Briefing Room to be opened immediately.

This mechanism, better known within Whitehall and to the media by its acronym of COBR, is an established part of the contingency machinery of government. It had been used to manage and coordinate responses to earlier civil emergencies, such as the fuel crisis in Autumn 2000. It would be deployed later in the year to respond to the terrorist attacks on the World Trade Centre and the Pentagon on 11 September 2001.

In activating the COBR mechanism on 22 March, the Cabinet Secretary requested that every available departmental Permanent Secretary should attend the first meeting, which he himself chaired at 1500 that afternoon. Ten Departments were represented along with the Scottish Executive and National Assembly for Wales. The Government's Chief Scientific Adviser was also present.

The participants went through the operational approach in place to eradicate the disease and looked at the available resources at each point of the process. In doing so, it became clear that the problem was not just lack of veterinary staff. The meeting agreed a series of actions to assess operational requirements in more detail and to begin levering in the wider resources of government. MAFF was to be asked each day whether any additional resources were needed. If any were, these would be provided at once. From this day an integrated strategic and operational response to the disease emerged.

COBR met twice daily until 5 April. The frequency of meetings was then reduced. A brief summary of its operation and functions during the FMD outbreak is set out in paragraphs 2.3.24-2.3.28 of the Government's Memorandum to this Inquiry (see the CD-ROM annexes).

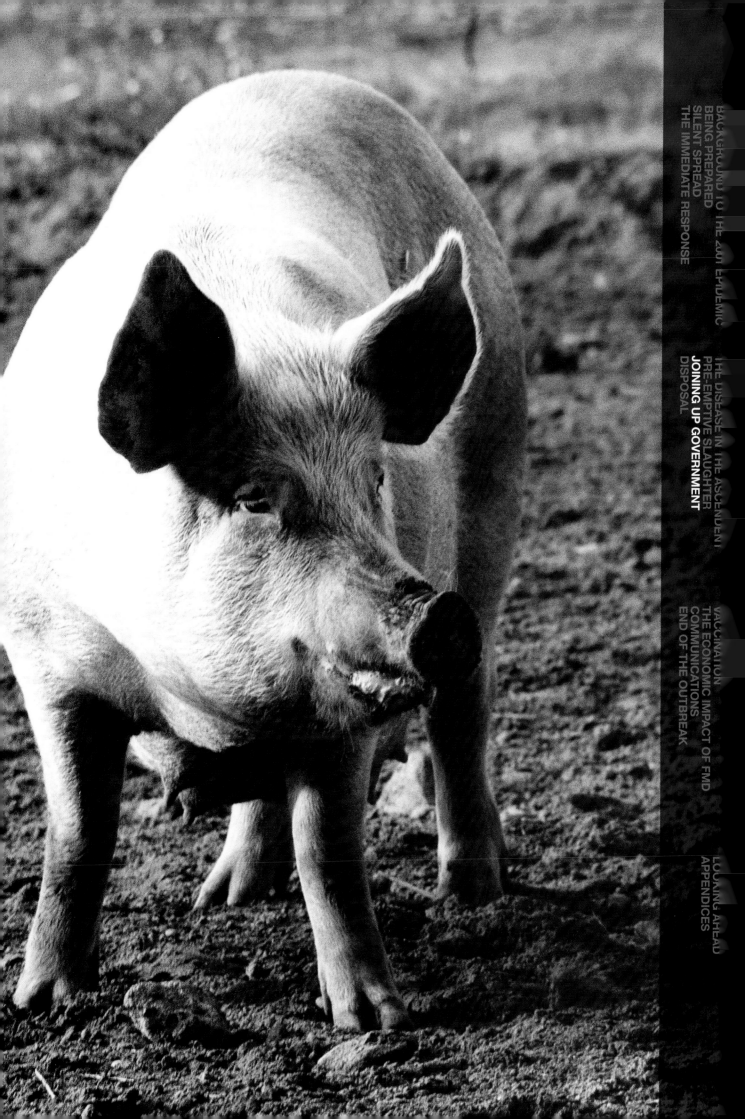

BACKGROUND TO THE 2001 EPIDEMIC
BEING PREPARED
SILENT SPREAD
THE IMMEDIATE RESPONSE

THE DISEASE IN THE ASCENDENT
PRE-EMPTIVE SLAUGHTER
JOINING UP GOVERNMENT
DISPOSAL

VACCINATION
THE ECONOMIC IMPACT OF FMD
COMMUNICATIONS
END OF THE OUTBREAK

LOOKING AHEAD
APPENDICES

"We all knew about speed, speed, speed and from where I was sitting … the main thing holding it up in the first six weeks was a fascination with an election date."

*Public Meeting,
regional visit to the South West*

11.2 Timing of COBR

The opening of COBR was a significant turning point in efforts to co-ordinate disease control activities on the ground and to mobilise logistical support across government.

From this moment and for several weeks thereafter, the Prime Minister took personal control of the crisis. And crisis it had become. Parts of the countryside were in chaos. Tensions inside and outside government were increasing. The epidemic was not 'under control' in any sense of the term. The COBR mechanism allowed the full force of government to be brought to bear. The goal was simple: to rid the country of the disease and to do so as quickly as possible.

Many submissions to the Inquiry suggested that government decisions at this time were heavily influenced by electoral considerations. The argument was that, in the first phase, a softly, softly approach was taken to avoid unnecessarily disturbing public opinion. Only when it became clear that this was not working was a heavy-handed approach adopted, again with an eye on forthcoming local and national elections.

We have examined government papers and questioned Ministers and officials but have found no evidence to support such a suggestion. Indeed, officials at all levels and in many locations are adamant that they were never exposed to any pressures other than the need to control the disease in the best possible way. Politicians would undoubtedly have had electoral considerations in mind, given the level of media speculation about the likely date of the General Election, but we have no evidence to support the notion that this had a significant bearing on policies or strategies for managing the disease.

Nor do we have any reason to doubt the Prime Minister's personal assertion that he was focussed entirely on tackling the disease. As a result of his preoccupation with the epidemic, delaying the local elections already set for 3 May and the General Election became inevitable. Electoral campaigns would have been impractical with the disease still rampant in large areas of the country.

Why then did it take 31 days from detecting the first case to putting in place the mechanisms and organisation that could bring to bear the full capabilities of government resources? These were 31 days during which a serious veterinary problem became a national disaster.

Part of the reason lies in the culture of Whitehall. Departments are often reluctant to seek help from each other. The outbreak was initially regarded solely as MAFF's problem. Without any formal review mechanism for reporting to the top of government, there was no structured way to challenge the prevailing view. There were, in short, no trigger points. There is a lesson here for the future.

39. **We recommend that a mechanism be put in place at the centre of government to assess potential domestic civil threats and emergencies and provide advice to the Prime Minister on when to trigger the wider response of Government.**

11.3 Management of information

We have already identified the issue of inadequate information flow. Put simply, those at the top responsible for major decisions were not provided with timely, accurate and relevant information about what was happening on the ground. Good management information systems and information analysis models would have shown, as early as the end of the first week of the outbreak, that existing resources were already stretched and in some parts of the country had been exhausted.

But, as late as 29 March, robust information on performance against the 24-hour slaughter target was still lacking. There were little data on disposal rates and a significant backlog of data on the operation of the 3km cull in Cumbria.

One of the earliest challenges for COBR was to improve the quality of management information it received from the ground. A note from the Permanent Secretary of the Cabinet Office to the Cabinet Secretary on 29 March (see CD-ROM annexes) set out the deficiencies in management information available to the centre and the steps being taken to rectify them.

The ability of the regions to enter data locally onto the Disease Control System at this time was, at best, limited. The bulk of the information was sent by phone, fax and email from the regions to Page Street where it was entered centrally. The fact that information came separately from Animal Health Divisional Offices and Regional Operations Directors made matters more complicated.

The Animal Health Divisional Offices had always collected data on the time of slaughter. They also recorded disease report times, although not until Saturday 24 March. The information was supposed to be passed to Page Street. But the severe pressure on resources meant that recording and reporting sometimes suffered, leading to backlogs and gaps. Where information was reported, it was not always made available to the local Regional Operations Director.

MAFF did not at first collect information on start of slaughter, a key parameter. Nor did its systems have the ability to measure properly performance against the 48-hour slaughter targets introduced on contiguous farms on 28 March. On 29 March, MAFF started collecting this information from Regional Operations Directors by telephone and entering the data at Page Street.

For the first two months of the outbreak – including the absolutely critical first three to four weeks – there was a serious deficiency in the reliability and completeness of the information available to those in charge of managing the disease.

"…you could see the colour drain from his [Jim Scudamore's] face when we were telling him. Jim Scudamore did not know, Nick Brown did not know, the communications blockage between what was going on on the ground and Carlisle, and then from Carlisle to Page Street, Page Street to the Minister, the Minister to the Prime Minister and the Cabinet, there were blockages all the way along."

*Public Meeting,
regional visit to the North West*

We believe that this lack of clear information on some of the most important indicators of the performance of disease control policies was a significant obstacle to managing the disease. There is a key lesson here for the future. The quality of management information in times of crisis is critical.

Whatever the contributory factors, MAFF Ministers and officials realised too late that managing the crisis was not only about securing sufficient numbers of vets – important though they were – but also about ensuring that other resources were available as well. Mechanisms within the Department had not been sufficiently sensitive to pick up the early warning signs that MAFF and the State Veterinary Service were being overwhelmed. The Prime Minister told the Inquiry that he was constantly asking MAFF whether they had sufficient resources to tackle the disease and was repeatedly assured that they thought they had. The reality, borne out by subsequent events, was different.

11.4 Reinforcing the crisis response

There was no mechanism at the centre of government to provide detached advice, at one step removed from efforts to tackle the disease, about when to reinforce the response to the crisis. DEFRA's Permanent Secretary told the Inquiry that such a mechanism would have served a valuable function. Neither the Cabinet Office nor the Home Office, the Department with lead responsibility for advising on domestic emergency planning arrangements at the time, fulfilled this role. This apparent vacuum in central advice and expertise on crisis management has subsequently been tacitly acknowledged by the creation of the Civil Contingencies Secretariat in the Cabinet Office following the General Election in June 2001.

The Civil Contingencies Secretariat will act, in future, as a trigger, alerting departments and the centre to potential problems across a range of issues. Its work will be based on horizon scanning and the assessment of information drawn from a variety of sources, both domestic and international. It will also advise departments on how to develop, rehearse and update their contingency plans. There is one essential caveat. The existence of the Civil Contingencies Secretariat must not reduce the incentive for departments to develop comprehensive contingency arrangements themselves.

11.5 Creation of the Joint Co-ordination Centre

The Joint Co-ordination Centre came into operation in MAFF on 26 March and was co-located with the existing Departmental Emergency Control Centre at Page Street. A brief summary of its operation and functions is set out in paragraphs 2.3.29-2.3.33 of the Government's Memorandum to this Inquiry:

○ Confirmed Cases

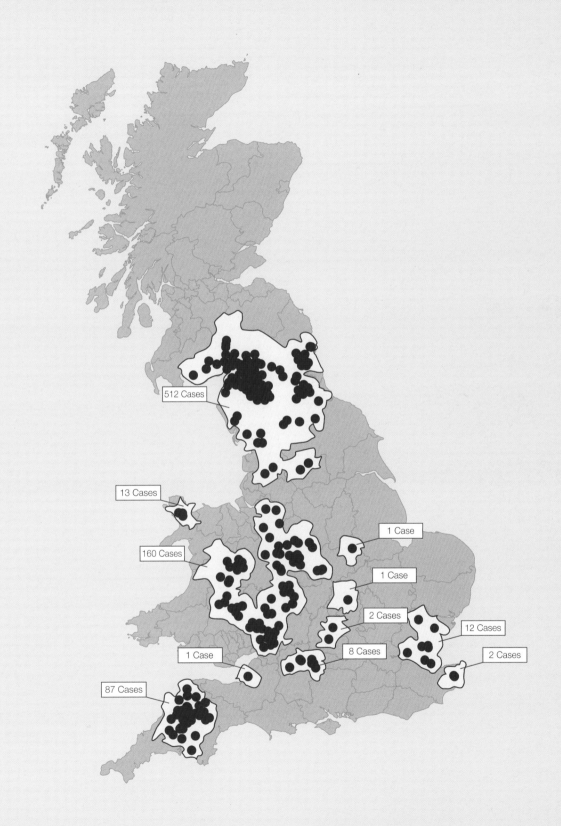

512 Cases

13 Cases

160 Cases

1 Case

1 Case

2 Cases

12 Cases

8 Cases

2 Cases

1 Case

87 Cases

"The function of the JCC was to provide and maintain an accurate ground picture of progress of the campaign, provide a liaison network to facilitate the rapid dissemination of instructions and information to the field and present information on the operation to all interested parties. It reported to COBR and to MAFF (later DEFRA) Ministers… It produced a daily report to COBR on the state of the epidemic, the resources deployed, the effectiveness of the operation, (the culling and disposal targets) disposal options, costs and on measures being taken to return the countryside to normality."

The Joint Co-ordination Centre benefited from the organisational and logistical expertise of the military personnel assigned to it, along with staff from other government departments. Thus the NFU wrote in its submission to the Inquiry: *"The military's role in the Joint Co-ordination Committee [sic] … proved to be a critical factor in achieving a more co-ordinated, applied and disciplined approach to tackling a wide range of logistical issues on the ground."* The NFU was represented in the Joint Co-ordination Centre to provide feedback on the impact of policies on the ground – an opportunity which was not extended to representatives of the wider rural economy.

40. We recommend that, in future, a representative of the wider rural economy be invited to participate in the Joint Co-ordination Centre.

Once they had been established and settled into a working pattern, both the Joint Co-ordination Centre and COBR made a significant contribution to the overall disease control strategy. At Cabinet on 29 March, the Minister of Agriculture reported that a huge effort was being made to bring the disease under better control and departments, especially the Ministry of Defence, had been most helpful in providing additional resources.

11.6 Handling of strategic and operational issues

Decision-making at a strategic level, involving the Prime Minister and the Minister of Agriculture, took place outside COBR. The Minister of Agriculture did not attend COBR. The Prime Minister has told us that, given the volume of work, responsibility had to be divided up. He decided that the Minister should lead on policy, keep the House of Commons informed and liaise with the farming industry while COBR dealt with logistics. It is not apparent, though, that this distinction was maintained throughout the crisis, or recognised by all those responsible for disease control activities on the ground.

Whether or not policy is decided inside or outside COBR, there should be well defined roles and functions at every stage of the process for managing a crisis. At a strategic level, the Prime Minister or Minister in charge must set the overall policy direction. At an operational level policy should be interpreted, parameters defined for action and appropriate resources made available. In our view, COBR and the Joint Co-ordination Centre fulfilled this function well. At a tactical level, those on the ground must understand what needs to be done and have the authority to do it.

In any crisis, especially one that mobilises the deployment of resources across Government, we perceive a need for detached, impartial advice at the most senior levels from individuals not directly involved in the emergency response. A 'senatorial group' whose membership would vary depending on the nature of the crisis could provide this. Such a body could give a valuable independent view on the handling of future national emergencies.

41. **We recommend that the concept of a 'senatorial group' be developed to provide independent advice to the Prime Minister and Cabinet during national crises.**

12.1 Introduction

Disposal of carcasses presented an enormous logistical problem. It created huge public concern and wide media interest. Images of mass burials and, particularly, huge pyres are still the emblem of the outbreak – even though the last pyre was lit on 7 May. While closure of footpaths may have been a major factor in keeping local tourists away from rural attractions, the images of the mass pyres, televised around the globe, undoubtedly kept away foreign visitors.

42. We recommend that burning animals on mass pyres is not used again as a strategy for disposal.

The issue of disposal and the inadequacy of provision for it had been noted in the Drummond Report in 1999 and further acknowledged by the State Veterinary Service in July 2000. The Dutch experience of disposing of nine million pig carcasses during the outbreak of classical swine fever in 1997 could have served as a warning for other countries to be prepared for a similar eventuality.

Contingency planning should have included consideration of a range of off-farm disposal options for various scenarios. It could have anticipated logistical problems that might arise from the location of disposal facilities, the size and species of animal, and the fact that many farms are accessed via narrow lanes. It should have drawn upon the Dutch experience and considered strategies to manage large scale disposal, such as vaccinating animals to postpone slaughter or freezing carcasses to pace the disposal. Better planning could have helped to reduce the backlog of carcasses and so improve the management of their disposal.

Disposal was an issue not only for the carcasses generated by disease control culling but also for the animals accepted onto the Livestock Welfare (Disposal) Scheme.

The Drummond Report commented that: "there is little time to debate the merits of one disposal method against another when disease has broken out and carcasses on the infected premises are starting to decompose." Yet this is exactly what happened in 2001.

The pre-existing Veterinary Instructions had a section on disposal of carcasses, predicated on disposal on the infected premises, preferably by burying, as recommended in the Northumberland Report. For disease control reasons moving carcasses off infected premises was best avoided.

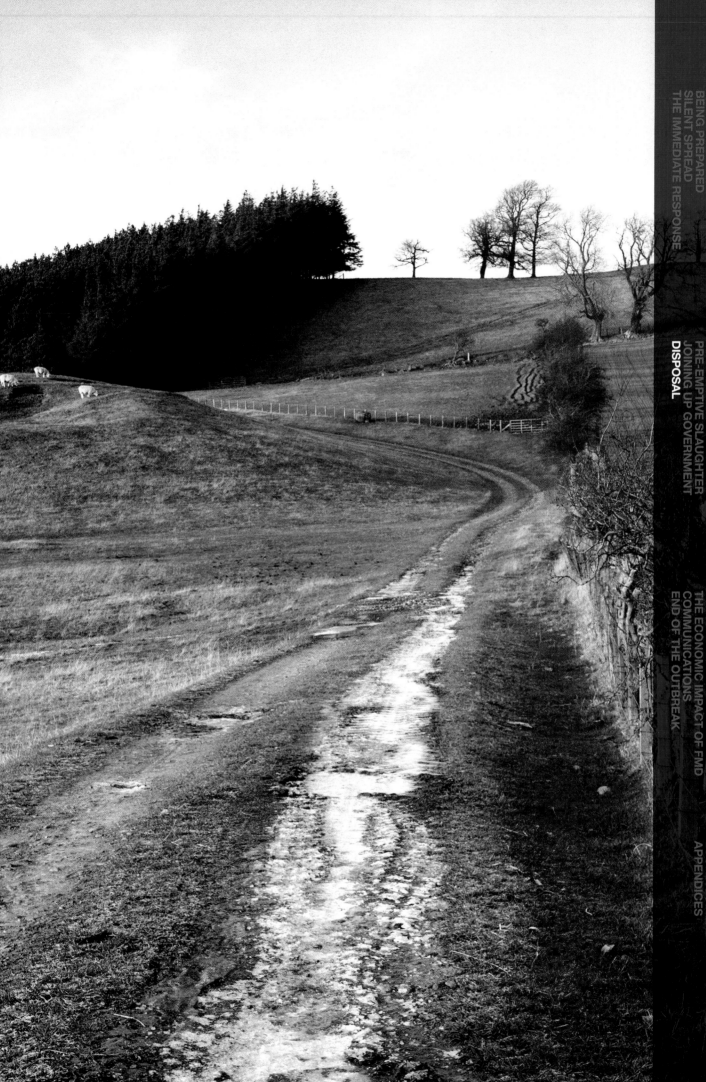

BACKGROUND TO THE 2001 EPIDEMIC
BEING PREPARED
SILENT SPREAD
THE IMMEDIATE RESPONSE

THE DISEASE IN THE ASCENDENT
PRE-EMPTIVE SLAUGHTER
JOINING UP GOVERNMENT
DISPOSAL

VACCINATION
THE ECONOMIC IMPACT OF FMD
COMMUNICATIONS
END OF THE OUTBREAK

LOOKING AHEAD
APPENDICES

From the environmental perspective, on-site disposal could create problems because of the potential contamination of groundwater. In the last major outbreak in 1967 this had been less of an issue. Awareness of environmental matters was less developed in 1967. The Environment Agency did not exist and legislation was less robust. Matters were aggravated in 2001 by an exceptionally wet winter and spring, with flooding and high groundwater levels. In addition, the records of the location of private water supplies were incomplete.

The Veterinary Instructions said that, where burial presented problems, burning was the alternative. A meeting between Ministers and the Chief Veterinary Officer on 21 February emphasised the need for swift slaughter and disposal, and agreed that "the most effective way of disposing of potentially large numbers of carcasses without putting public health at risk would be to burn them….(although) the environmental consequences would possibly need to be raised with the Environment Agency."

It was not long before the volume of carcasses was posing serious problems. Farms were much larger in 2001 than in 1967. Average herd and flock sizes had doubled (5.4.2). As a result, the logistics of disposal became more complex. For example, in Cumbria in the early weeks, four individual cases generated 1,458 cattle and 17,270 sheep for slaughter – and a further 15 dangerous contact farms to be culled. A pro rata calculation on these 15 dangerous contacts would give a total of some 90,000 carcasses linked to the four original cases.

12.2 Pressure builds

The option of rendering carcasses was first considered on 5 March. A Deputy Chief Veterinary Officer, at a veterinary management meeting, was charged with checking if there were any blockages in the slaughter and disposal chain, and whether there was a role for the military to help in containing the outbreak. The following day it was agreed to investigate the use of air curtain incinerators. On 10 March, it was agreed that off-farm disposal should be used in areas where narrow roads prevented transportation of burning equipment to the farm site. By 12 March, the Chief Veterinary Officer reported rendering to be running smoothly in Wales and Scotland but that, in Cumbria and Devon, there were real concerns about disposal.

The root of the problem was the weight of numbers. At this time, there was a view that this would not be solved by military intervention, although the possibility of extending pre-emptive culling and hence increasing the number of carcasses made it worth considering the role the military could play. The decision to request military vets from the Ministry of Defence was taken on 14 March. The first military logistical deployment occurred in Devon on 19 March.

Between 15 and 30 March six possible sites for mass burial were identified (Ash Moor in Devon, Great Orton in Cumbria, Birkshaw Forest in Dumfries and Galloway, Throckmorton in Worcestershire, Eppynt in Powys and Widdrington in Northumberland). A seventh site, Tow Law in County Durham, was added on 5 April, after burial had commenced at all the others except for Ash Moor which was never used.

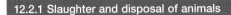

12.2.1 Slaughter and disposal of animals

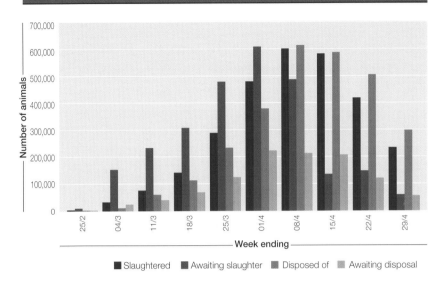

The backlog of slaughtering and carcasses awaiting disposal is shown in chart 12.2.1. By 1 April, at the peak, 622,000 animals were awaiting slaughter and 230,000 were awaiting disposal.

12.3 Public health and environmental impact

From a disease control point of view, the disposal of carcasses had, if necessary, to be dealt with separately from slaughter even though this resulted in carcasses lying on the ground for some time. Dead animals excrete much less virus than live ones.

The standing Veterinary Instructions contained guidelines on disinfecting and monitoring carcasses awaiting disposal. Carcasses were disinfected, but close monitoring of carcass heaps was not routine. There were fears that heaps of carcasses could contribute to disease spread by rats. There is a small theoretical possibility that such transmission could occur.

Later on in the outbreak, on 21 June, the Secretary of State for Environment, Food and Rural Affairs, Margaret Beckett, said that the Department of Health had advised that the greatest hazard for public health would result from leaving carcasses out in the open.

The public health aspects of disposal, other than those associated with groundwater, were only belatedly considered. The Department of Health was not routinely represented at the Joint Co-ordination Centre in the early phase. Not until 24 April did the Department of Health issue guidance on minimising the risks to public health. There was the added complication of the possibility of BSE in cattle over 30 months old. The existing FMD Veterinary Instructions did not address this. Record keeping early in the outbreak was poor, so the age of cattle buried or burned at a given location was not always known. Policy was developed during the first weeks of the outbreak and some disposal sites were retrospectively assessed. The Spongiform Encephalopathy Advisory Committee made a recommendation on the disposal of pyre ash in May 2001.

Several organisations were responsible for aspects of environmental and health control (12.3.1). Local authorities were responsible for air quality near pyres, use of commercial landfill, and private water supplies, but they were not actively involved by MAFF early enough, nor systematically. In some regions local authority officers have told us that the Regional Disease Control Centre seemed unaware either of the legal responsibilities of local councils or at which tier of local government responsibility lay.

43. We recommend that training for those with responsibility for managing disease control include the relevant legal frameworks and the structure and responsibilities of local government.

44. We recommend that all agencies with responsibility for public health be actively involved in designing disease control strategies and in contingency planning and communications.

The Environment Agency had developed a risk-based hierarchy that identified rendering and high temperature incineration as the preferred options. However, rendering capacity was limited and not conveniently located. There were a few high temperature incinerators capable of taking whole cattle carcasses, but these were already fully committed. By the end of the outbreak the summary disposal statistics in England and Wales were as shown in 12.3.2.

In Scotland, 98% of carcasses from infected premises were burnt on-farm. The remainder were rendered. The majority of other Scottish animal carcasses were buried at Birkshaw Forest.

The risks to the environment and public health associated with disposal have been shown to be minimal. There were 212 water pollution incidents, only three of which were classified as 'major' incidents. The majority of incidents, including the three classified as 'major', were associated with problems of disposal of slurry arising from movement restrictions.

12.4 Mass burial and landfill

By 10 May the problem had been overcome. The disposal backlog had been reduced to 350 by a combination of military logistical support and the creation of mass burial sites.

Mass burial sites generated significant opposition from local communities who were concerned about possible environmental damage and risks to health. Fears were aggravated by the fact that the concept of mass carcass burial was new and hence the design of the sites was novel. There were also concerns that the transport of infected carcasses into the area could, of itself, spread the disease. Such concerns were not allayed by leaking wagons which were seen on some occasions. We have not found any evidence that this was a mechanism of spread but, at the height of the outbreak when emotions were high and the stress on rural communities immense, the uncertainties associated with disposal did not reassure local people.

12.3.1 Organisations with responsibility for environmental and public issues

Issue	Lead organisation
Government policy and legislation affecting the environment	Department for Environment, Food and Rural Affairs (DEFRA) Scottish Environmental Protection Agency National Assembly for Wales Department of Health
Air pollution i.e. noise, smoke, smell problems Environmental health	The local authority (except when they relate to a site at which the Environment Agency regulates emissions to the air)
Planning permission	The local planning authority
Contaminated land	The local authority (but sometimes the Environment Agency will have a lead role)
Supply of public drinking water	The local water company
Monitoring of quality of private drinking water supplies	The local authority
Sites of Special Scientific Interest and nature reserves	English Nature
National Parks	The appropriate National Park Authority
Rights of way and access to the countryside	Countryside Agency
Drinking water quality	Drinking Water Inspectorate (public supplies)

Source: Information supplied by Environment Agency North East Region, Northumbria Area

12.3.2 Summary disposal statistics

Disposal method	Provisional statistics	Comment
Burning (on farm)	Over 950 sites	Based on available DEFRA/National Assembly for Wales data for England and Wales.
Burial (on farm)	900 sites	DEFRA/National Assembly for Wales estimate for England and Wales.
Mass burial	61,000 tonnes at four sites	DEFRA/National Assembly for Wales estimate for England and Wales to August.
Commercial landfill	95,000 tonnes at 29 sites	Environment Agency estimate for England and Wales to September.
Rendering	131,000 tonnes at seven plants	DEFRA/National Assembly for Wales estimate for England and Wales to October.

Source: Environment Agency, December 2001

> "The people of Tow Law were presented with a *fait accompli* on the evening of 6 April at 2 hours notice, the public meeting had 2 hours notice. That, Sir, is a disgrace, it is a total contempt of any kind of stakeholder involvement."

Public Meeting,
regional visit to the North East

The speed with which decisions were taken, from site selection to construction and use, meant that there was little or no time for consultation. In many instances, Environment Agency groundwater authorisation was given retrospectively. In one case, Eppynt in Wales, the paucity of existing geological information and the lack of time for a thorough site investigation meant that the authorisation proved to be inappropriate and the site had to be closed.

The lack of consultation angered local communities who were not always told of the plans before work had commenced. Local MAFF officials were left with a difficult community liaison task to manage over the following weeks and months. One front line official explained how protesters squirted her with liquid they claimed was leachate, and dumped chopped liver on her car. Such incidents appear to have been rare. Protest was strong but generally peaceful.

Mass disposal sites still remain a contentious issue even with the passage of time. They appear to have blighted the communities nearby. They cost significant sums of money to maintain and monitor. The National Audit Office report on the 2001 FMD outbreak contains further financial details.

Commercial landfill could, in theory, have accommodated all the stock slaughtered for disease control purposes and via the Livestock Welfare (Disposal) Scheme, thereby removing all the costs of construction and ongoing management associated with the mass burial sites. Of the 111 landfill sites identified as suitable only 29 were used, taking 95,000 tonnes of carcasses. Few landfill operators were willing to accept carcasses. In the face of this reluctance, driven largely by public and local authority opposition, the Government would have had to direct the individual landfill licence holders to take carcasses. The risks of being directive were seen to be too great. This problem could have been avoided if planning for mass disposal had been undertaken and standby arrangements with landfill operators put in place in advance.

We believe that much anguish could have been avoided and resources could have been saved had disposal been given due consideration during the period following the Drummond Report. There are lessons here for the future.

Open and honest communications with local communities at such times of tension are vital. Decisions about mass disposal would never have been popular, but the lack of information and perceived insensitivity to local concerns aggravated the situation. In addition, local communities that eventually accommodated a mass burial site, received no compensation from the Government at all. Such a payment might have gone some way to mitigating the distress felt by those in local communities.

45. **We recommend that local communities be consulted on mass disposal sites according to best practice guidelines, and that the question of compensation for communities accommodating emergency disposal sites be researched. We recognise that this is a complex legal area nationally and at EU level.**

12.5 Role of the Environment Agency

The Environment Agency's links with MAFF at the outset were not good. The Agency reported to us that they had to press to get involved in some regional centres. Where on-farm burial was occurring, the Agency did desk-based assessments of the proposed site, as far as possible with a three-hour turn around time. They also carried out assessments of the proposed mass burial sites. They were able to draw upon a variety of data sources and the local expertise of their area based staff. This approach was satisfactory where the data available were robust. But there were sometimes errors in the grid references supplied to the Agency for on-site burial. There were limited data on the exact source of private water supplies. In Wales, the geological database produced by the British Geological Survey was not sufficiently complete to make reliable assessment for mass burial.

12.6 Cleansing and disinfection

Once carcasses had been disposed of, farms had to undergo cleansing and disinfection before restrictions could be lifted. The National Audit Office FMD Report contains a detailed case study on cleansing and disinfection and the associated costs which accords with the picture we have established.

A major complaint presented to us was that the delay in completing the cleansing and disinfection process, and the associated delay in removing restrictions, not only had adverse implications for the farmer, but also added to delays in reopening footpaths.

We were also told how cleansing and disinfection was sometimes undertaken by contractors who had little or no knowledge of farms or farming. There was no standard approach to follow because the structure of farms varied widely. Different contexts presented different cleansing problems. The National Trust, for example, experienced difficulties when inexperienced contractors and officials attempted to apply inappropriate cleansing strategies for listed buildings.

A water company in the North East explained to us how failure to involve them in planning and on-going discussion came close to creating a local water incident. Huge volumes of water were drawn from the network for cleansing and disinfection.

12.7 The Livestock Welfare (Disposal) Scheme

The need for some form of welfare scheme had been apparent early in the epidemic. The movement and trade restrictions, particularly in Surveillance and Protection Zones, were likely to lead to welfare problems if they extended for any length of time.

During the classical swine fever outbreak in 2000 MAFF had had to introduce a welfare scheme for pigs, not principally because of movement restrictions but because of the absence of a market for susceptible animals. That scheme had been administered by the Intervention Board, a body whose main responsibility was intervention in the Common Agricultural Policy. The Intervention Board had disposed of over 180,000 pigs during the classical swine fever outbreak. The staff in MAFF and the Intervention Board who had experience of the classical swine fever scheme were asked early in March 2001 to draw up a similar scheme for the FMD outbreak.

The principle behind the classical swine fever scheme had been that it was a scheme of last resort. It was expected that farmers would want to retain their animals if at all possible. Initially the scheme had only offered free collection and disposal. Pressure from the farming industry resulted in the introduction of payments which eventually reached about 70% of the animals' value. The industry itself topped up the payments (via a £4 million Government loan repaid by levy).

In designing the scheme for FMD, MAFF was anxious to avoid such a negotiation of rates. So, in striking a balance between the principle of a scheme of last resort and the desirability of buy-in from the farming industry at the outset, the proposed Livestock Welfare (Disposal) Scheme rates were set at around two-thirds of market value and notified to the EU, as required by law, on 16 March.

However, on 22 March, at a meeting at Number 10 attended by the Prime Minister and the English and Welsh Ministers for Agriculture, representatives of the farmers' unions in England, Wales and Scotland arrived to negotiate the payment rates. The English Minister for Agriculture and his officials had anticipated pressure from the unions. He had been prepared to move the average level of compensation up to 70% but this was less than the unions were asking for. The Minister and his officials expressed concern that higher rates would create an alternative market. In the event, the meeting agreed the Minister's proposal in relation to pigs and hoggets but also agreed the unions' proposals of 90% for breeding animals and 80% for clean cattle. The scheme was announced later that day with these increased rates.

Those who had developed and were to run the scheme, but who had not been present at the Number 10 meeting, knew that the increase in rates would attract far greater participation in the scheme than had been planned for. The scheme became a first port of call rather than a last resort. It was soon deluged, and outstripped the capacity of the Intervention Board to handle claims.

One aspect of the last resort design was that it would not require any veterinary input to check and prioritise applications. Farmers would only apply if in real need and with the support of their local vet. The generous nature of the scheme that was negotiated, encouraged applications in cases that were not yet serious or not even genuine welfare cases.

The Intervention Board did not have the resources or expertise to manage prioritisation and verification. At the start of the outbreak it only had one vet. It later had three vets. Later still the RSPCA provided valuable input to prioritising cases on strictly welfare grounds.

Matters were made worse because the Livestock Welfare (Disposal) Scheme had been designed, sensibly, so as to slaughter only when the disposal route was clear, and to use spare rendering capacity. Yet on the day after launch all spare rendering capacity had been commandeered to deal with FMD culled animals. Furthermore the outbreak was spreading and so were the associated restricted zones, generating still more welfare problems.

The Intervention Board had picked up the administration of this scheme at a time when it was on the brink of a large-scale reorganisation and was in the process of developing major new computer systems. The organisation had no regional structure yet the FMD outbreak was being regionally managed. The Livestock Welfare (Disposal) Scheme was a paper-based system. It was unable to cope from the outset with the scale of take up.

Pressure on the Livestock Welfare (Disposal) Scheme was a recurrent theme in situation reports to the Joint Co-ordination Centre and COBR over the following weeks:

"Huge backlog of cases. Intervention Board appear to be totally overwhelmed by the size of the problem. The scheme is simply not working".

"The Minister heard about the difficulty of contacting the Intervention Board. Consideration should be given to increasing the capacity of the helpline."

"The blockage was in disposal. Until landfill or rendering capacity could be unlocked... the scheme was effectively stalled".

At Inquiry meetings around the country regular reference was made to the inadequacies of the Livestock Welfare (Disposal) Scheme. The numbers were so large and the ability to deal with them so small. For example, in Wales twice as many animals were slaughtered on welfare grounds as were for purposes of disease control.

The blockage on disposal continued as it proved difficult to negotiate access to commercial landfill for disposal of welfare carcasses. *'There is already confusion on the ground, hostility and suspicion and increasing local authority action or threat of action to halt the process. In some cases the co-operating landfill contractors are being strong armed or threatened with suspension of other contracts to prevent them from taking this waste. There needs to be much more of a high level communicate and persuade exercise'* (Status report to Joint Co-ordination Centre/COBR 4 April 2001).

Disposing of unpleasant waste attracts public opposition at the best of times. In the midst of the FMD crisis the public had little sense of the distinction between diseased and welfare carcasses. There were concerns about all types of disposal. Trying to persuade landfill companies, local authorities and the public to accept carcasses against this backdrop was bound to be very difficult. When landfill capacity was successfully contracted prices were up to ten times those in normal circumstances.

One third of the applications to the scheme came from Wales, but there had been only limited landfill available in Wales so most of these animals were disposed of in England. The location of disposal facilities supports the case for retaining a national rather than a devolved approach to disease management.

Applications to the scheme were handled by the office of the Intervention Board in Newcastle, and then passed to the Board's office in Reading for slaughter and disposal arrangements to be made. The volume of applications, limited numbers of staff, inexperienced staff on helplines and the absence of a computerised system with any linkage to other farm databases all contributed to delays in processing. There were duplicate entries in the system, representing 876,000 animals. An improved database system eventually helped to detect and eliminate them. This duplication, combined with last minute withdrawals, was at the root of problems such as contractors arriving to slaughter only to find that the job had already been done or was no longer needed.

The RSPCA played a valuable role in assisting with local welfare problems and in pressing for prioritisation of urgent cases. They also contributed to avoiding welfare problems on the ground by supplying many tons of fodder and bedding and, on occasion, tents for lambing.

There were numerous instances of severe welfare problems and long delays. Some animals died before arrangements could be made for slaughter. However we have heard, from many quarters, that some farmers took advantage of the scheme and disposed of healthy animals. The RSPCA provide a case study in their submission in which they observe that the animals in question were worth around £50 per head but would have been valued at £81 by the Scheme. The National Audit Office reported that, in early April 2001, COBR noted that payment levels were providing incentives to farmers to let their livestock become welfare problems. Livestock Welfare (Disposal) Scheme rates were revised downwards in late April and again in late July following review and consultation. A related scheme for light lambs was introduced on 3 September and, given a longer lead in time and fewer animals, ran more smoothly.

No contingency plan for any large-scale welfare disposal scheme existed. The scheme was conceived and developed during the early weeks of the outbreak and the last minute nature of it, coupled with the rise in payments in response to farming pressure, rendered much of the planning useless as it undermined key design principles of the scheme. DEFRA's interim FMD contingency plan of March 2002 has not addressed welfare issues.

The welfare scheme whose design had worked in the classical swine fever outbreak, would probably have come under strain, even without the last minute increase in rates. In the different context of FMD, the duration and geographic spread of the disease made the prospect of sale of potential welfare cases in future markets less likely. The extensive and extended nature of the outbreak created more welfare cases than anyone would have predicted and put pressure on limited disposal resource. Farmers have told us that very limited movements, strictly for welfare reasons, ought not to be incompatible with disease control so long as they are subject to strict biosecurity controls. This warrants consideration in our view.

46. **We recommend that the Government consider the welfare implications of disease control policies, as part of contingency planning for FMD and other diseases, and seek to identify strategies that minimise the need for slaughter and disposal on welfare grounds.**

13.1 Vaccination

Vaccination was one of the most hotly debated, yet misunderstood, aspects of the FMD epidemic. Our Inquiry concentrated on policy matters surrounding vaccination, while the Royal Society Inquiry examined the scientific issues.

The debate about vaccination in 2001 has to be seen in the specific context of animal vaccination. There are two aspects to this: disease control and the implications for international trade.

Vaccination can be used in different ways to control an FMD outbreak (13.1.1). The UK considered the use of emergency vaccination during 2001. It never considered routine mass vaccination of all animals against FMD.

13.1.1 Vaccination terminology	
Routine (or prophylactic) vaccination	• Mass vaccination for long-term prevention when FMD is endemic or recurrent. • Not permitted within the EU.
Protective vaccination	• Emergency vaccination of a limited number of animals in a restricted area ('vaccination to live').
Suppressive vaccination	• Emergency vaccination and subsequent slaughter of a limited number of animals in a restricted area ('vaccination to die').

13.2 International Animal Health Code

Different disease control strategies have different implications for international trade and regaining disease-free status, as described in the International Animal Health Code of the international organisation, the OIE (13.2.1) and discussed in section 14.3. The Code sets the standard for the World Trade Organisation. However, individual member countries decide how to incorporate the rules into their own national arrangements.

The International Animal Health Code had not, until May 2002, explicitly taken account of the use of emergency protective vaccination in which vaccinated animals were allowed to live out their normal economic lives. The disease status of countries which vaccinated their animals, but did not subsequently slaughter them, was not clear. In particular, the period that countries using emergency protective vaccination had to wait until they regained 'FMD-free without vaccination' status could have been 12 months, two years or longer, depending on how the Code was interpreted.

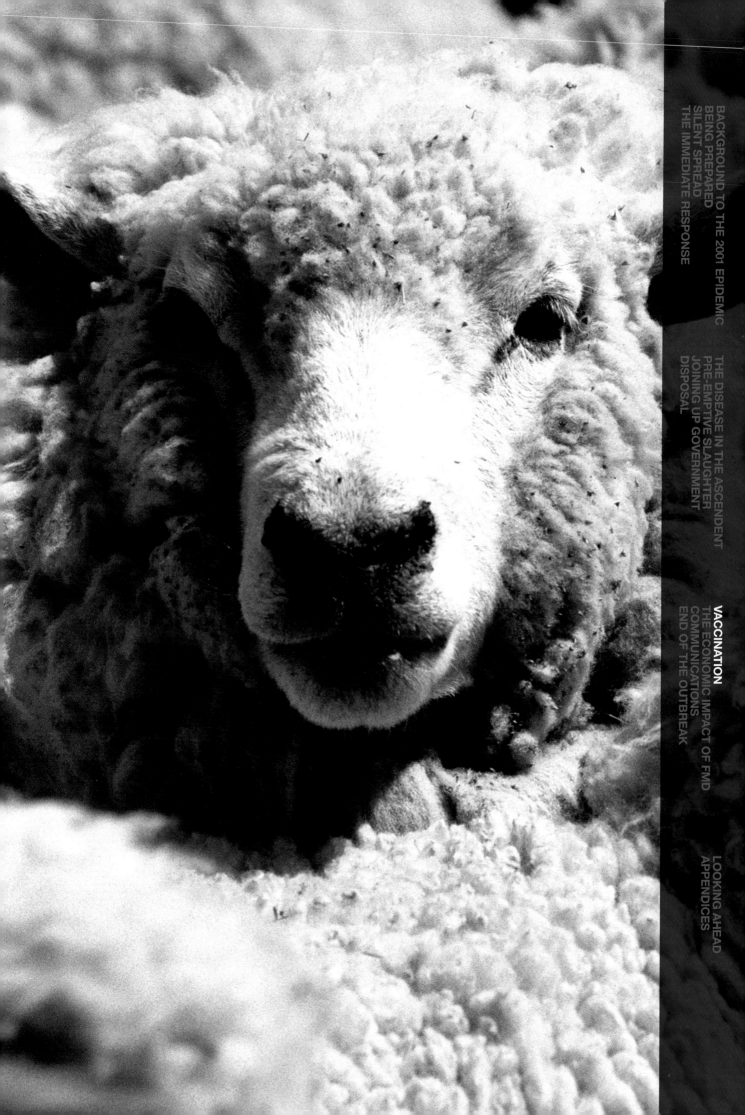

13.2.1 International Animal Health Code in 2001

FMD-free country without vaccination	• No outbreak for the past 12 months
	• No vaccination for at least 12 months
	• No importation of vaccinated animals since the cessation of vaccination
FMD-free country with vaccination	• No outbreak for the past 2 years
	• Routine vaccination with a vaccine complying with the OIE standards
	• System of intensive surveillance for detection of any viral activity

FMD-free zones require surveillance or buffer zones, or physical or geographical barriers that separate the free zone from the infected territories.

The Code stated:

When FMD occurs in an FMD-free country or zone where vaccination is not practised, the following waiting periods are required to regain the disease-free status:

a) 3 months after the last case where a stamping-out policy and serological surveillance are applied, or

b) 3 months after the slaughter of the last vaccinated animal where stamping-out, serological surveillance and emergency vaccination are applied.

When FMD occurs in an FMD-free country or zone where vaccination is practised, the following waiting periods are required to regain the disease free status:

a) 12 months after the last case where stamping-out is applied, or

b) 2 years after the last case without stamping-out, provided that an effective surveillance has been carried out.

The International Animal Health Code was revised at the OIE General Session in May 2002 (13.2.2). It is now more explicit about the conditions regarding status. Countries using emergency protective vaccination can regain their disease-free status after six months, provided they test for non-structural proteins (NSP) in continuing serological surveillance (16.3.1). The reduction in time decreases the impact on exports, making the use of vaccination more acceptable.

NSP tests, developed over the last few years, are a variation on the antibody ELISA tests used in serological surveillance. Although now included in the International Animal Health Code, NSP tests have not been validated and their precise application in the field has yet to be determined.

13.2.2 Revised International Animal Health Code May 2002

When an FMD outbreak or FMD virus infection occurs in an FMD-free country or zone where vaccination is not practised, one of the following waiting periods is required to regain the status of FMD-free country or zone where vaccination is not practised:

a) 3 months after the last case where a stamping-out policy and serological surveillance are applied, or

b) 3 months after the slaughter of the last vaccinated animal where a stamping-out policy, emergency vaccination and serological surveillance are applied, or

c) 6 months after the last case or the last vaccination (according to the event that occurs the latest), where a stamping-out policy, emergency vaccination not followed by the slaughtering of all vaccinated animals, and serological surveillance are applied, provided that a serological survey based on the detection of antibodies to non-structural proteins of FMD virus demonstrates the absence of infection in the remaining vaccinated population.

One key issue in the vaccination debate in the UK was how to discriminate between vaccinated and infected animals. Those opposing vaccination were concerned that vaccinated animals might transmit infection without showing signs of disease. Advocates of vaccination, on the other hand, argued that the NSP tests could be used to resolve that problem.

All viruses, including the FMD virus, are made up of proteins. These proteins can be structural or non-structural. Infected animals produce antibodies against both. However, vaccinated animals produce antibodies against structural proteins only. A positive NSP test detects antibodies against non-structural proteins and therefore identifies an infected animal.

13.3 EU Policy

The EU holds the highest status of 'FMD-free without vaccination'. This permits Member States to export animals and meat to any country in the world. As part of preparation for the single European market in 1993, the EU decided to harmonise its approach to vaccination. Previously, most Member States used routine vaccination to prevent outbreaks of disease. The exceptions were the UK, Ireland, Greece and Denmark.

The EU conducted a cost-benefit analysis of disease control strategies (14.4). The benefits of a stamping out policy outweighed those of mass vaccination campaigns because the frequency of FMD outbreaks in the EU had decreased over the years. Accordingly, the routine use of FMD vaccines was prohibited and Member States phased out vaccination between 1991 and 1993 following provisions contained in amending Council Directive 90/423/EEC (5.4.4).

> "Ten years after vaccination was brought to an end in Europe the debate that it provokes has not lost any of its intensity. Its supporters and its opponents confront one another in a dialogue in which the certainties on one side are matched only by the confidence on the other."

French Senate Inquiry Report into FMD 2001, Chapter IV: III (English translation)

Although routine vaccination is no longer an option for EU Member States, the International Animal Health Code permits FMD-free countries to use emergency vaccination in the event of disease outbreaks. A Member State can only use emergency vaccination with the approval of the EU Standing Veterinary Committee. In 1999, the European Commission Scientific Committee on Animal Health and Animal Welfare adopted a report entitled 'Strategy for Emergency Vaccination against FMD'. It contained guidelines, including criteria to aid decision-making related to protective vaccination, and recommended that contingency plans should provide estimates of the total number of vaccine doses required.

By 2001, therefore, the use of vaccination to tackle an FMD outbreak anywhere in Europe was subject to European law. No Member State could act unilaterally. In the event of an outbreak, each country needed to consider its response in the light of the European legal framework.

In the UK, the initial policy approach was not to use vaccination but to rely on the traditional stamping out policy. The Netherlands, by contrast, with its large export market, opted for suppressive vaccination. This involved implementing a planned vaccination programme, developed in the wake of the 1999 classical swine fever outbreak, followed by slaughter of vaccinated animals. The strategy meant that disease-free status could be regained three months after slaughter of the vaccinated animals when exports could resume. It allowed a more orderly process for slaughter and disposal, although some have argued that more animals were culled than might have been had stamping out alone been implemented. The numbers culled – 267,992 animals on 2,763 affected premises for 26 infected premises – led to public criticism of the policy.

13.4 Contingency planning for vaccination

We found no evidence that the UK took heed of the 1999 European report guidelines in altering UK strategic policy. Contingency planning for vaccination was minimal.

Instructions for vaccination were prepared in the Veterinary Instructions. The version available at the start of the outbreak had been produced in May 1998, and provided an outline procedure. It recognised that the existing legislation was out-of-date and required revision in light of EU Directive 85/511 (5.4.4).

In a report prepared for the Inquiry, the Chief Veterinary Officer wrote, on 28 March 2002, that: *"No estimate has been made of the human resource requirements for a vaccination programme. For the purpose of this paper the assumption is made that a stamping out policy would be operated first and that, if sufficient trained resources were immediately available as outlined, vaccination could be avoided."*

Plans for vaccination during the FMD outbreak had to be developed at the same time as fighting the disease.

13.5 Proposed vaccination of cattle in Cumbria

Vaccination was considered within the first week of the outbreak, but generally thought to be impractical. Nevertheless, a flurry of activity ensued. MAFF commissioned papers from experts, such as scientists at the Pirbright Laboratory, and information was gathered urgently. They concluded that, due to the widespread nature of the infection, vaccination would have little to contribute to disease control at that stage. The scientific and practical pros and cons of vaccination options and their implications for trade should have been thought through in advance of the outbreak.

At a meeting on 12 March, the Prime Minister was content with the decision not to vaccinate and it was recorded that the Chief Veterinary Officer *"noted that some people were advocating vaccination as a viable alternative strategy. However, he saw a number of insurmountable difficulties with it, not just in terms of disease control but in terms of the UK's ability to export meat and livestock, and the negative impact on UK tourism. He believed it very unlikely that the EU would press us to introduce a vaccination programme."*

The disease picture continued to worsen from mid-March onwards. Daily numbers of cases continued to rise. On 19 March, the Chief Veterinary Officer visited Cumbria and decided that a plan of action was urgently needed in case vaccination were required. Cattle that had been housed over the winter were to be released to spring pasture over the following weeks. The density of infection in sheep in Cumbria was such that dairy cattle were at great risk if they were let out before the infected sheep had been culled. Options were considered and cost-benefit analyses conducted. With the State Veterinary Service already fully stretched, ADAS Consulting Ltd was engaged on 23 March to draw up operational plans for a vaccination programme.

Vaccination in Cumbria was considered primarily as a means to protect cattle from the disease and allow them to live out their normal economic lives. The aim was to reduce the numbers of cases and release resources for other priorities.

Within the proposed vaccination zone, control measures required by the EU would have had practical implications for food production, such as milk pasteurisation and treatment of meat products. The Government did not plan to pay compensation, even though EU law provides for partial reimbursement of Member States for any compensation paid for losses incurred as a result of post-vaccination controls.

Vaccination was discussed by the FMD Science Group many times throughout the epidemic. From their first formal meeting on 26 March, most of their early meetings dealt with vaccination and the use of models to predict its impact on disease control. On 10 April, the Group unanimously recommended vaccination of the housed cattle in Cumbria, providing that it did not detract from the slaughter and disposal operations, and that co-operation from the farmers was secured. They advised that it would not reduce the spread of the disease but would prevent the loss of many valuable animals, and that the decision must be taken quickly since delays would decrease the benefit.

MAFF made the necessary preparations. On 27 March, it recommended to the Prime Minister that, *"a programme of emergency vaccination of cattle should be undertaken as a matter of urgency."* Authorisation from the EU Standing Veterinary Committee was applied for on the same day. It was approved and then adopted on 30 March. 500,000 doses of high potency vaccine (O1 Manisa strain) were available from the International Vaccine Bank at the Pirbright Laboratory. 156 vaccination teams recruited by ADAS Consulting Ltd were put on a three-day standby. Nothing happened.

13.6 Lack of support for vaccination

For all the urgency, discussions were still taking place with industry groups. The farmers' unions were neither convinced of the scientific rationale nor the need for vaccination, given the implications for export markets. Furthermore, support would depend on assurances that the food industry would accept products from vaccinated animals.

The food industry was nervous that consumers would not buy food products from vaccinated animals (13.6.1), despite the Food Standards Agency's assertion that there were no health risks. The issue came to a head at a summit meeting called by the Prime Minister at Chequers on 12 April. It was Maundy Thursday, the day before the Easter weekend. This was a critical time for the tourist industry. The disease was still raging. The number of daily cases had fallen to around 30 per day from the peak of 50 recorded on 30 March. Much of the country was still under strict movement controls. On 2 April, the Prime Minister had postponed local elections planned for 3 May.

In a note of the meeting at Chequers, the Prime Minister had summarised the situation: *"The NFU remained strongly opposed to vaccination. But they also said that this opposition depended in large part on fears that the retailers would shun the products of vaccinated livestock. If the industry decided that it would accept the products, farming opinion could shift quite quickly."*

The farmers' unions remained resolutely opposed to vaccination throughout the crisis. Vaccination was postponed when the Cumbrian farmers agreed to keep their cattle housed for longer to allow time for the risk to be removed by culling the infected sheep in the area. In fact, the 3km cull in Cumbria was resisted and only partially completed. On 18 April, the Government announced that vaccination was still being considered and that industry views were being sought. But, without the full co-operation of farmers, a vaccination campaign could not have been effective. By the following week, the reasons for vaccination were less compelling. The cattle had been let out and the epidemic was in decline. The plans for vaccination in Cumbria were abandoned.

Vaccination was seriously considered on several occasions. However, the decision to vaccinate as an additional control measure was overshadowed by the lack of support on the ground.

13.6.1 Consumer attitudes to FMD vaccination

The decision on whether to vaccinate animals against FMD relied, in part, on the anticipated reaction of consumers to food products from vaccinated livestock. Surveys throughout the crisis gave equivocal answers. A definitive view could only have been gained by testing consumer behaviour in the marketplace.

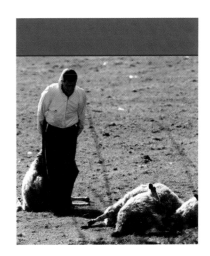

The Food Standards Agency made clear, both at the Prime Minister's meeting with the food industry on 12 April and in its announcement on 27 April, that products from FMD vaccinated animals posed no additional risks to food safety, in the same way that produce from livestock routinely vaccinated against other diseases can be consumed without concern. Consumer organisations concluded that it was unlikely to be an issue for consumer choice and therefore that products would not require special labelling. The Soil Association and organic producers supported this view.

Despite these assurances, some parts of the food industry had worries about consumer confidence. They feared that vaccination would generate a two-tier market. Consumers might demand labelling and have a preference for other sources of produce, such as imported meat. The consequences of the decision on vaccinating cattle in Cumbria were made clear by the Prime Minister when he met the food industry, as recorded on 12 April: *"if the case for vaccination were rejected by the industry, the result could be the slaughter of a large part of the dairy herd. The public might respond very negatively to this, and to the fact that the situation had come about because of resistance to vaccination by the farming and food industries."*

Surveys conducted by the Institute of Grocery Distribution revealed two main areas of concern and confusion for consumers: the indecision over the use of vaccination and the motives behind the livestock cull. Most consumers preferred vaccination to slaughter. Some consumers believed that products from FMD vaccinated animals were safe but still preferred not to consume them.

13.7 Vaccination re-visited

The vaccine stocks held at the Pirbright Laboratory reached their expiry date at the end of May 2001, but commercial supplies of vaccine were delivered (1.5 to 3 million doses per month) until January 2002 and stored at the Merial UK site, next door to the Pirbright Laboratory, on behalf of DEFRA.

In May, the Settle outbreak and general disposal problems led to vaccination again being raised at COBR meetings. The outbreak in Thirsk in July also prompted DEFRA to consider vaccinating cattle in that area. However, in each case, vaccination was rejected.

Some special cases for vaccination were considered carefully but also rejected. For example, it was decided not to vaccinate rare breeds or hefted sheep. Some breeds represent rare genetic stock which cannot easily be replaced, although ova and semen can be stored in gene banks. Hefted sheep result from years of careful breeding during which knowledge of the parcel of land, the 'heft', is passed on from ewe to ewe lambs. As part of the policy adjustments announced on 26 April, rare breeds and hefted sheep were exempted from the contiguous cull provided that strict biosecurity was maintained.

Following appeals from hefted sheep farmers and others to vaccinate their animals, the Foot and Mouth Disease (Control of Vaccination) Regulations 2001 were introduced on 5 July. These prohibited vaccination without a licence from the Secretary of State as the disease free status of the whole country or defined zone would have been affected by the use of vaccination.

Proposals to vaccinate hefted sheep on the Brecon Beacons in Wales were considered in depth during July. The pros and cons were assessed, including the contribution to disease control, the costs and the economic impact on agriculture and tourism, and practical issues of implementation. COBR advised against vaccination, but considered how the culling policy might be modified if the disease proved to be much more widespread than the initial epidemiological analysis suggested. In the event, a major programme of blood-testing confirmed the initial epidemiological analysis. Further culling was not needed.

The final major consideration of vaccination started towards the end of July, when the dense pig farming areas in Humberside would have been at risk had the disease spread eastwards from the Thirsk area. If the pig farms had become infected, FMD could have spread widely because pigs excrete large amounts of airborne virus. Options for the pre-emptive vaccination of pigs and cost-benefit analyses were considered against various assumptions. None of the risk scenarios transpired, although DEFRA Ministers made clear to the Inquiry that the potential impact on disease control was so great as to override all doubts about vaccination.

13.8 To vaccinate or not to vaccinate

To vaccinate or not in various locations and at various times created considerable controversy during the epidemic. The issues were complex, even for professionals with relevant clinical experience. The UK was not well prepared. Policy decisions and practical issues had not been thought through in advance. Attempts to work out strategies with interest groups at the height of the crisis caused confusion in the minds of the public and led to delays in taking clear decisions.

Several opportunities for protective vaccination were considered in detail in association with EU officials. There were many conflicting points of view. Even when the science was clear, the practicalities and economics were not. Co-operation from the farming community as a whole was not achieved, and the concerns voiced by some sectors of the food industry about public acceptability of vaccinated products strongly influenced the decision not to vaccinate cattle in Cumbria.

47. We recommend that the Government establish a consensus on vaccination options for disease control in advance of an outbreak.

There are important conclusions to be drawn from these experiences.

- Emergency vaccination must form part of the strategic options available to manage any future outbreak.
- DEFRA should maintain an appropriate state of readiness, together with a shared understanding in the EU and among stakeholders, of the conditions where vaccination will be used.
- Export restrictions must be based on sound scientific evidence so that economic penalties are minimised.
- The farmers' unions and other parties must engage with DEFRA to deliver this goal.

48. We recommend that the Government ensure that the option of vaccination forms part of any future strategy for the control of FMD.

49. We recommend that the State Veterinary Service maintain the capability to vaccinate in the event of a future epidemic, if the conditions are right.

"…science appears to have let us down, our industry did not have a suitable diagnostic test, nor had the debate on vaccination been conducted suitably between 1967 and the present outbreak, they had had plenty of time. That debate should have been conducted, the situations under which vaccination might have been used ought to have been clearly relayed to us all and then it would have saved a lot of the nonsense and debate that did go on."

Public Meeting, regional visit to Scotland

14.1 The Government's estimate of the impact of FMD on the economy as a whole

The 2001 Pre-Budget Report[1] estimated that the impact of the FMD epidemic on the country's Gross Domestic Product, or GDP, was less than 0.2%, equivalent to nearly £2 billion. But, the impact on GDP is likely to be much less than the true costs of the disease.

This is because the GDP effect only measures the resulting loss of output. Some costs such as the human ones discussed below are not included at all and the loss of value of livestock is not captured properly. Furthermore, the resources employed in treating the disease and managing its consequences, whilst counting as production in the calculation of GDP, are resources which in the absence of the disease would largely have been productively employed elsewhere in the economy.

Although, losses to sectors directly affected by the disease were, from a macroeconomic perspective, largely offset by increased spending elsewhere, the impact on tourism in the affected areas was devastating. Some of that activity was diverted to other UK locations and to consumer spending on unrelated items. This reduced the effect on total output. It did not, however, reduce the severe costs that were imposed on or within particular sectors. Some consumers also suffered because they would have preferred to spend their money in the countryside but were unable to do so, and this is not captured by GDP.

It is, however, correct to measure the losses which resulted from FMD by the effect on value added in the producing sectors. Some high figures have been cited as a result of using gross revenue, before deducting the costs associated with that output or considering alternative uses. In particular, the costs associated with export restrictions are not the value of the exports affected, but the value of the exports less their cost of production, or the value of exports less the value which would be derived in lower value uses.

The Government has estimated the net costs on the sectors or types of businesses most adversely affected. These were agriculture and the food chain, together with those businesses directly affected by tourist expenditure. These estimates were published in a joint paper by DEFRA and the Department of Culture, Media and Sport[2]. The paper shows how rural and urban areas were affected and assesses the regional impact. The impact on the wider rural economy is considered in section 9.11 of our report. While most of the effects will have occurred in 2001 some of the agriculture effects are likely to be felt for a number of years.

---

[1] Pre-Budget Report 2001, HM Treasury, CM5318.

[2] The Costs of Foot and Mouth Disease in the UK; joint paper by DEFRA and Department of Culture, Media and Sport, 2002.

All the estimates are limited by the nature of the available information. The impact on domestic tourism is subject to serious data limitations and has consequently drawn heavily on survey data. So cost estimates for businesses directly affected by tourist expenditure are presented in broad ranges.

Agriculture

The main costs in this sector resulted from the slaughter and disposal of livestock, either to control the disease directly or to deal with animal welfare problems. The Government compensated farmers for their loss of livestock by some £1.34bn. This figure includes compensation for any infected materials seized or destroyed.

During the crisis, professional valuers determined the value of the animals for compensation purposes. The average compensation for cattle rose from around £500 in the early weeks of the outbreak to a peak of around £1500 in May, before falling back to around £1200 in September. The average compensation values for sheep rose from an initial £100 to £300 in July and then also declined. A standard rate card was introduced in March 2001. To encourage its use the standard rates were based on the upper quartile of market prices before the February outbreak. The rates ranged from £150 to £1100 for cattle and £32 to £150 for sheep.

In some cases, it is likely that the compensation paid to farmers exceeded the amount which they would have expected to obtain for their animals in normal conditions, possibly by substantial amounts. It was judged necessary to pay farmers on a generous basis to ensure their co-operation in the slaughter policy. The costs of this represented a transfer of resources from taxpayers at large to the farming community.

The outbreak imposed other costs on this sector (14.1.1). These were estimated at £355m on agricultural producers. Some £175m was incurred as a result of the restrictions on animal movements.

Farmers within or close to infected areas, whose farms were subject to Form D restrictions suffered greatly. They incurred the costs of keeping animals and were subject to strict movement controls. However, they received no compensation.

Food chain

There were further costs imposed on the food chain; most markedly on auction markets, slaughterhouses and food processors. These activities were disrupted by the movement and export bans. The Government estimates that the total loss of value added for these sectors was some £170m.

14.1.1 Sectoral Economic Effect of FMD (Agriculture, Food Chain and Tourism) 2001- 2005

Sector –		£ million
Agricultural producers		-355
of which:	Market prices[1]	-50
	Export loss[2]	-130
	Withholding costs[3]	-175
	Consequential costs[4]	-35
	Sheep Annual Premium[5]	-120
	Agrimoney aid	+155
Food Industry		-170
of which:	Auction Markets	-95
	Abattoirs	-40
	Processors/hauliers	-35
Tourism[6] (range)		-2700 to -3205
Indirect effects		
Agriculture/food chain[7]		-85
Tourism[8] (range)		-1835 to -2180

[1] Market prices represents a loss of revenue associated with price changes consequent upon the changed pattern of marketings.

[2] Export loss is an additional effect associated with lower quality domestic uses (e.g. pet food) for supplies diverted from export.

[3] Withholding costs are the extra costs and deterioration in quality associated with holding animals on farm beyond optimum marketing dates.

[4] Consequential losses are those associated with the loss of production whilst farms are prevented from re-stocking.

[5] Sheep Annual Premium/Over Thirty Months Scheme/Agrimoney are associated subsidy changes, some of which are co-funded by the EU budget.

[6] Losses of gross value added.

[7] Additional (indirect) costs.

[8] Estimates from input-output multipliers to all industries linked to tourism.

Source: DEFRA and the Department of Culture, Media and Sport

> "…it is a tragedy that an animal illness has been translated into one that had severe impact on the mental health of our patients."
>
> *GP, Devon*

Tourism

Overall, the tourist sector, both rural and urban was estimated to have lost between £2.7 and £3.2bn of value added in 2001 as a result of FMD. Within these figures there were winners and losers. Some businesses only a few miles apart from an FMD outbreak were affected in very different ways. Some were hardly affected or even have had increased business, while others were forced to close.

Differential effect on rural and urban areas

The costs for agriculture, food and tourism were disaggregated to derive estimates of the differential impact on rural and urban areas. The loss in rural areas was in the range £2.2 to £2.5bn, while the loss in urban areas was in the range £0.8 to £1bn. The vast majority of these costs related to reduced spending on domestic tourism.

Regional impact

The Government also derived regional estimates of the costs to agriculture and the food industry. Approximately two thirds of the costs occurred in England, with around one sixth each in Scotland and Wales.

Indirect costs

The industries which supply agriculture, the food industry and tourist related businesses, also suffered. The aggregate effect on these industries was estimated at £1.9 to £2.3bn. Within this, the overall impact on suppliers to the agriculture and food industries was a relatively modest £85m because FMD led to increases in the demand for some types of input, such as feed, as well as reductions in demand for other inputs. It was not possible to derive rural or regional estimates for these indirect costs.

Public sector

In addition to £1.34bn in compensation for the losses associated with livestock slaughter, the Government met other costs linked with the outbreak. These are set out in table 14.1.2. Total costs to date to the public sector were £2.8bn.

Although some farmers were compensated for the vast majority of their losses, businesses affected by reduced tourist expenditure received little compensation.

14.2 Human and other costs

The above figures relate only to those effects that have proved relatively easy to measure. The outbreak also had further impacts, including the stress caused to farmers and others, restrictions on access to the countryside, health effects and environmental costs

In many areas affected, the social structure and sense of community were severely damaged. There was often little social contact as many were confined and unable to go about their usual life.

14.1.2 Expenditure on FMD by Government[1]

Activity	Actual Expenditure to 24 May 2002 (£ million)
Payments to farmers	
Compensation paid to farmers for animals culled and items seized or destroyed	1,130
Payments to farmers for animals slaughtered for welfare reasons[2]	211
Total payments to farmers	**1,341**
Direct costs of measures to deal with the epidemic	
Haulage, disposal and additional building work	252
Cleansing and disinfecting	295
Extra human resource costs	217
Administration of the Livestock Welfare (Disposal) Scheme, including operating costs, disposal charges and slaughter fees	164
Payments to other Government departments, local authorities, agencies and others	73
Miscellaneous, including serology, slaughterers, valuers, equipment and vaccine	68
Claims against the Department	5
Total direct costs of measures to deal with the epidemic	**1,074**
Other costs	
Cost of government departments' staff time	100
Support measures for businesses affected by the outbreak[3]	282
Total other costs	**382**
Total costs	**2,797**

[1] All costs are provisional pending completion of a DEFRA project to investigate the full costs of the outbreak.

[2] Includes payments of £205.4 million under the Livestock Welfare (Disposal) Scheme and £5.3 million under the Light Lambs Scheme.

[3] Includes money available under European Union market support measures for agri-monetary compensation in respect of currency movements.

Source: DEFRA, NAO

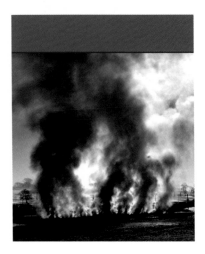

14.2.1 Haydon Bridge High School

Haydon Bridge High School in Hexham, Northumberland, serves the local community with 750 pupils coming from a 700 sq km catchment area. It has a boarding house for 50 weekly boarders. There is also a School Farm, on site, with beef and dairy cattle and sheep.

Many pupils come from farming families and so, coupled with the farm on site, the school had a unique insight into the effects of the outbreak.

In the early days, the only way to make appropriate decisions was through information gathered in consultation with other schools, forming a partnership of 19 schools in Northumberland, and through a local NFU representative who happened to be a school Governor. Communications from either County Hall or DEFRA invariably came by post so they were already out of date on arrival. Often they were inconsistent. County Hall's advice on disinfectant mats was that they should be banned for health and safety reasons. DEFRA, on the other hand, insisted on their use if the school wanted to have its Form D notice lifted in early September and be open for the autumn. The Form D has been placed on the school and its farm in late August, as the Hexham hotspot raged. Neither the school nor the farm was told that this had happened.

Early in the epidemic, on Friday 2 March, 40% of students (286) were absent. With exams approaching, the school found itself in a very difficult position: how to maintain the education of its students, while at the same time maintain biosecurity on the farms?

"By now (3-4 March), all of the community is within a restricted area. A whole swathe of students, and six staff could be absent for weeks rather than days. This is confirmed by even more phone calls and by reference to the Internet. How ironic that information travels fast; many of our students not at all. How frustrating that our long-standing pleas for improved I.T. facilities in this most rural area have often fallen on deaf ears. We still have to use the post to send work home – and to receive urgent messages from County Hall."

The school and its Ridley Hall boarding home had the added burden of a financial cost due to the outbreak. The £10,000 bill was first sent to County Hall and then on to DEFRA. As of the end of May 2002, the school had not received any payment.

During our Inquiry visits, we heard many examples of poor communication, all of which led to increased stress and mental hardship for the local populations.

Many members of the public were denied access to, and hence enjoyment of, the countryside. Government officials also suffered in trying to manage the epidemic.

We received a number of submissions regarding the perceived health risks from mass pyres and the disposal sites. These issues were raised by North Cumbria's director of Public Health in his submission to the Cumbria Inquiry into FMD. He felt strongly that the Department of Health should have been brought in earlier to advise on such matters and to reassure the public.

In addition to the human or health effects, there were also environmental impacts resulting from the disease control measures, most notably those associated with carcass disposal. These are discussed further in section 12.

Although such costs were often difficult to measure, they remain legitimate components of an overall assessment of the effects of animal disease control strategies, and should be taken into account in decision making.

50. **We recommend that Government make explicit the extent to which the wider effects of disease control strategies have been identified, measured and taken into account in policy decisions.**

14.3 The benefits of FMD control strategies

The financial costs of the 2001 epidemic mostly fell on those outside the farming community: taxpayers at large, other businesses related to agriculture and, most importantly, other businesses in rural areas. Many farmers were substantially compensated for the financial costs of the epidemic: others were not. The human costs in terms of stress and isolation did however fall disproportionately on farming families and rural communities. It is reasonable to ask what was gained in return for all these costs, both those that were possible to measure, and those where measurement was much more difficult.

The benefits of FMD control accrue to farmers, rural communities and society as a whole. In addition to maintaining exports of livestock and livestock products, benefits include lower costs of livestock production, better animal health, maintaining foreign tourism, and avoiding constraints on UK travellers abroad.

The total livestock and livestock products export market was worth £2,343.4m and £1,314.7m in 1995 and 2000 respectively (14.3.1). As a result of the ban on exports, some products intended for export were diverted to the domestic market, albeit possibly sold at lower prices or as inferior products.

"There are children out there in our schools now we are still giving counselling to, they are still traumatised and will continue to be so."

*Public Meeting,
regional visit to the North West*

The ability to maintain these exports is significant for those engaged in the agricultural export trade. From a national economic perspective, however, the value of maintaining exports of £1.3bn is not material in relation to the total costs incurred in controlling the 2001 epidemic.

But failure to control FMD would substantially increase the costs of UK livestock production; possibly by such an amount as to make a large proportion of current livestock production unviable.

On narrow economic grounds, it is difficult to see why costs as substantial as those of the 2001 epidemic should be met by people not engaged in agriculture. In most industries, in which there is a possibility that a failure within the industry will impose substantial costs on people outside the industry, there is an expectation that the costs of failures will mostly be met by the industry concerned.

We accept that it is neither possible nor acceptable that the farming industry should bear the full costs associated with that control. There are wider benefits of controlling FMD, which accrue to the country as a whole. The implication of this is that the public should bear at least some of the costs of maintaining a healthy and extensive livestock industry. But, in return, the farming industry must recognise that it, along with others, has responsibilities for the rural economy and should contribute to its future development.

14.3.1 The livestock and livestock products export market

Exports (£m)	1995			2000		
	EU	Non-EU	Total	EU	Non-EU	Total
Beef and veal	540.1	60.1	600.1	20.4	0.6	21.0
Pig meat (excl bacon & ham etc)	200.3	45.3	245.7	127.7	38.4	166.0
Ham etc.	15.1	1.2	16.3	20.2	1.1	21.4
Live pigs	29.7	5.8	35.5	12.4	0.7	13.1
Sheep meat	307.5	6.4	313.8	198.0	3.8	201.8
Live sheep	106.0	0.0	106.0	72.0	0.0	72.0
Milk/milk products	611.7	184.5	796.1	466.1	167.9	634.0
Poultry	191.6	38.2	229.9	156.6	28.8	185.4
Total	2,002.0	341.5	2,343.4	1,073.4	241.3	1,314.7

Source: DEFRA

We therefore support the position of the Policy Commission on the Future of Farming and Food. The way ahead for agriculture, including animal disease control, must be seen in the context of an overall strategy for the rural economy in which the agricultural sector is but one of a number of interests. In the heat of the 2001 epidemic, policy was driven mostly by the urgent needs of the agricultural sector. In longer term planning for future contingencies, a wider range of interests must be considered.

51. **We recommend that the interests of all the sectors likely to bear the brunt of any costs be properly represented and taken into account when designing policy options to control animal disease outbreaks.**

14.4 Cost benefit analysis of FMD control strategies

A comprehensive cost-benefit analysis of the 1967 outbreak[3] concluded that the economic benefits of FMD control exceeded the costs of control, whether through slaughter or vaccination, by a substantial margin.

However, a full scale updating of the costs and benefits of controlling FMD was not carried out. Such an updating is overdue. A number of factors is likely to have changed since the 1960s. For example, tourism has grown in significance both in terms of GDP and employment. The values that society places on, for example, the environment and avoiding the unnecessary suffering of animals is unlikely to be the same now as it was some 30 years ago.

52. **We recommend that cost-benefit analyses of FMD control strategies should be updated and maintained. These should be undertaken at both the UK and EU level.**

[3] A Cost-Benefit Evaluation of Alternative Control Policies for Foot and Mouth Disease in Great Britain, Power A. P., and Harris S. A., MAFF, 1973.

15.1 Introduction

Good communications are essential to any organisation's business. The same applies to government. In times of crisis government has a special responsibility to communicate clearly and accurately to the population at large.

Throughout the work of our Inquiry, 'communications' was a recurring theme. It touched, and sometimes enraged, many people affected by the epidemic.

This section summarises how the Government communicated, what others did and what more could be done to ensure that communications are well targeted and effective should a serious animal disease break out. As the DEFRA director of communications said to the Inquiry: "If there is an information vacuum, then mis-information and myth creep in."

15.2 The principles of good communications

The guiding principle for government in a crisis is to explain policies, plans and practices by communicating with all interested parties clearly and consistently in a transparent and open way. This should be done quickly, taking account of local circumstances.

The elements that underpin that guiding principle are as follows:

- be honest and open;
- ensure the facts are right;
- correct any mistakes as soon as possible;
- provide information that is up-to-date;
- provide as much local or regional detail as possible;
- tailor information to different audiences;
- communicate internally as well as externally;
- make maximum use of available technologies;
- be inclusive;
- communicate promptly.

These are useful yardsticks by which to assess the capacity and flexibility of any communications system during a crisis. While some were practised during the FMD epidemic, others were not.

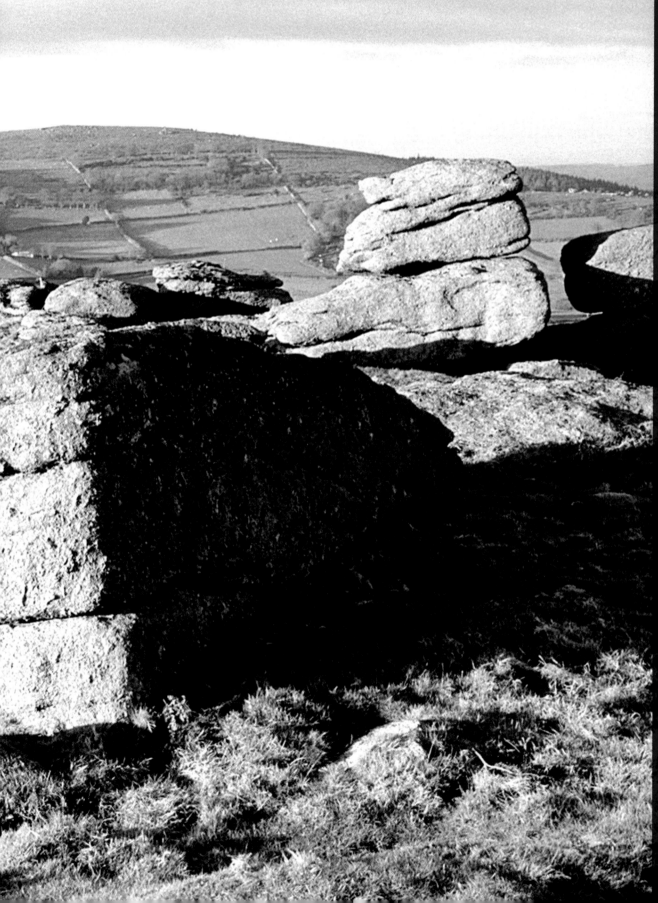

15.3 The national response

When the first case of FMD was diagnosed on 20 February 2001, MAFF's press office had a small staff and no regional structure. It did not immediately reinforce its numbers nor set off an emergency response. It was, understandably, not geared up to the 24 hours a day, 7 days a week routine that crisis management demands. There were no trigger mechanisms to alert MAFF to the potential for increased demand on its communications resources. Only from the weekend of 24-25 February did such measures start to be put in place.

In the early hours of any crisis, speed and clarity of communication matters. Just as with tracing the spread of FMD, so presenting a clear message about the nature of the disease is critical.

53. **We recommend that the Government build into contingency plans the capacity to scale up communications systems and resources rapidly at the onset of any future outbreak of animal disease.**

54. **We recommend that a government-wide crisis communication strategy be developed by the Civil Contingencies Secretariat with specific plans being prepared at departmental level; for example by DEFRA and the devolved administrations in Scotland and Wales in the context of animal disease control.**

As the disease spread, MAFF put in hand a number of initiatives. A website was opened on day one and updated thereafter. Daily briefings led by the Minister of Agriculture and the Chief Veterinary Officer were started on 21 February. These briefings gave a factual account of the spread of the disease. Journalists to whom we spoke said how much they welcomed them. Much of the early press coverage was factual and positive. For example, on 23 February, The Times described the Government as having acted with "exemplary speed". The following Monday 26 February the Sun said of Nick Brown, the Minister of Agriculture, that "he has acted with calm authority quickly making the right decisions while avoiding creating an atmosphere of panic".

As the crisis deepened, daily briefings become more of a burden than a benefit. The Head of the Pirbight Laboratory said that preparation for media interviews took up a disproportionate amount of his time.

Face-to-face daily media briefing is not essential in a crisis. What is vital is that accurate information is provided quickly and is easily accessible.

On 25 March 2001, the daily MAFF briefings were discontinued. National press briefing came from Number 10 and the Cabinet Office. Media briefings should add value and information. The twice daily political lobby briefings by Number 10 made little sense when there was nothing new to say and briefing political journalists made less sense than briefing specialist journalists, some of whom felt excluded. This was particularly so at the time of the development of the contiguous cull.

15.4 Communications with stakeholders

The weekly stakeholder meetings set up by MAFF every Friday were valuable. The first of these was on the first Friday of the outbreak, 23 February. They continued on Fridays throughout the whole crisis.

Participants at these meetings told us how useful they were. However, dissemination of information from those meetings was inconsistent. Some stakeholders got information onto their websites quickly. The Food and Drink Federation showed us examples of the electronic briefing notes sent to all their members within hours of the close of stakeholder meetings. By contrast the Department's website was sometimes not updated quickly. This caused confusion.

MAFF regional offices and local government frequently received information informally via local stakeholders, before they received it officially. Sometimes, when regulatory changes were made, local officials were not given enough warning. This caused confusion among farmers and others seeking information.

Local helplines were established. But operators were overstretched and did not have enough up-to-date, detailed knowledge. In some cases, local offices took on support from the local NFU or used voluntary helpers to deal with the large number of callers. We were told that, at the start of the crisis, many Disease Control Centres were unable to deal with offers of help from local communities.

Information was not fully co-ordinated on a national and local scale. COBR meetings did not have consolidated management information for the purposes of overall strategic management of the crisis (9.3 and 11.3).

55. **We recommend that DEFRA develop its regional communication strategy and ensure that it has effective systems for disseminating clear and concise information quickly to all its regional offices. This should be developed in the context of cross-government crisis management planning, in consultation with the Regional Co-ordination Unit and Government Offices.**

"About 10 days after the cull on our farm we received a letter [from DEFRA] saying because of foot and mouth infection all the livestock on your farm has been culled. ... did they think we were asleep and we hadn't noticed?"

Public Meeting,
regional visit to the North West

Communications with regional stakeholders are important. DEFRA's internal communications systems should disseminate facts rapidly to its local offices. Local staff must be able to access that information. Computer systems should be robust enough to deliver this.

15.5 The role of new technology

The MAFF website was opened on day one of the crisis.

The Government's Memorandum to the Inquiry stated that the official website was "the most direct source of information on the outbreak for farmers, the public and the media." However, some journalists and members of the public told us that the website was often out of date. Farmers in Cumbria told the Inquiry that, when the website was obviously out-of-date or inaccurate, they rang the helpline but got no better information. Staff on the helpline drew their information from the website. So, if the website was out-of-date, so was the helpline.

The Internet is an important tool. It can only be effective if the information presented is timely and accurate. As more and more farmers get access to the Internet, its potential for communicating in a crisis will increase.

56. **We recommend that DEFRA resource its website to ensure it is a state-of-the-art operation. In any future outbreak, the website should be used extensively, and a central priority should be to ensure that it contains timely and up-to-date information at national and local level.**

15.6 Direct communications

Over the course of the epidemic the Department sent out 16 mailings including a video on biosecurity. The Disease Control Centres also sent out information directly. For example, the Exeter Disease Control Centre alone sent out over 30 information sheets.

It has been difficult to assess the value of these mail shots. We were told that they were often ineffective. By the time some of the mail shots were read, they were already out-of-date.

Some of the routine disease notices were poorly written. The Animal Health Act (1981) Form D notices, which put farms under a movement standstill, have been widely criticised in our public meetings and in meetings with individual farmers for being poorly written and lacking clear explanatory notes.

57. **We recommend that DEFRA commission research into the effectiveness of its direct communications during the FMD outbreak of 2001 so that all the lessons may be learned, acted upon and the results published.**

58. We recommend that the State Veterinary Service revise all its
disease control Forms A-E and information about exotic animal
diseases in liaison with the Plain English Campaign.

15.7 The regional and local media

FMD affected different areas in different ways. The pattern and size of
disease spread varied enormously. At one end of the scale Cumbria had
over 40% of all outbreaks. At the other end Northamptonshire had only one
case. Local communications should reflect such differences.

The regional media during the epidemic fulfilled a special role. They were
always on hand, pressing the local agenda on what they saw as a London-
imposed national agenda. The Western Morning News, Western Daily
Press, The Journal (Newcastle), Northern Echo, Yorkshire Post, News &
Star, Cumberland News, The Scotsman and Dumfries & Galloway Standard
and others saw clearly how the national crisis was affecting their local
communities.

There were media campaigns on local issues, especially the issue of
disposal. Local stories often became national headlines, none more so than
Phoenix the Calf (15.7.1).

MAFF was slow to strengthen its regional media capacity. Initially it relied
too much on local staff who had no media training or background. As it
became clear that they would not be able to cope, the local Central Office
of Information became more involved. Regional Operations Directors,
appointed in mid- to late March, took over co-ordination of local
communications.

A section of the media that received widespread praise in the course of our
Inquiry has been local radio. It provided the vital service of telling local
people what was happening and where in their locality. At its best it was
up-to-date, accessible and regularly available. In Devon, BBC local radio
station provided twice daily programmes at set times giving updates on all
aspects of FMD. In Cumbria, BBC radio broadcast updates seven times
a day, five times in the morning and twice in the afternoon. In Yorkshire,
BBC North Yorkshire split its frequencies and broadcast special news
updates in the morning, at lunchtime and in the early evening.

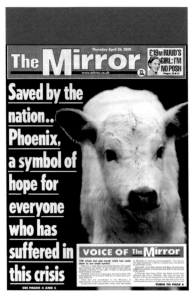

Source: The Mirror

15.7.1 Phoenix the Calf

The Charolais-cross calf Phoenix was born in Devon on Friday 13 April, Good Friday. Her herd was culled five days later. When the disposal teams arrived to remove the carcasses, Phoenix was found unharmed. The media called for her to be saved. These appeals reached a peak around 24 and 25 April. On 26 April, the contiguous cull policy was refined and Phoenix's life was spared.

The Government firmly denied that Phoenix had influenced its policy change. The decision to change policy had been made some days before Phoenix came to the nation's attention. It had already been arranged that the Minister of Agriculture, Nick Brown, would make a statement explaining the policy change in the House of Commons on 26 April.

However, on the evening news bulletins of 25 April and in The Mirror the next morning, the implication was that policy had been changed specifically in order to save Phoenix. We do not believe this to be so. In evidence to the Inquiry the Prime Minister's Director of Communications and Strategy said that *"we [Downing Street] agreed with MAFF on the 25th that the Phoenix story was becoming a real distraction, and that, as Nick's statement would have the coincident effect of sparing Phoenix, that should be communicated to the media. This was during the evening of April 25th in time for the late bulletins. This did not pre-empt the statement, other than to say that Nick Brown would be making this statement, and it would be clear from what he said that the individual circumstances of the likes of Phoenix would be taken into account."* (See CD-ROM annexes.)

In any future outbreak, the local media should be used to the full. DEFRA should provide tailored information to local radio stations or local newspapers in time for their deadlines, working with the Government Office network and the Government News Network. Similar arrangements should be made in Scotland and Wales.

Central government should consider how best it can support and strengthen regional communications in times of crisis. Regional Operational Directors responsible for local communications should be trained in media skills.

15.8 The international media

The international media was prominent throughout the crisis, viewing the epidemic from a different standpoint from the national and regional media.

Pictures of mass pyres spread around the world. Tourists chose not to visit a burning Britain. As far as the outside world was concerned, Britain was in the grip of yet another animal plague: it was not only unhealthy to eat British food – it was also unwise to visit Britain.

59. **We recommend that communications strategies during a crisis take special account of the needs of the international media.**

16.1 Biosecurity

Biosecurity entered the farming vocabulary during 2001. Few people were familiar with the concept at the start of the outbreak. It involves measures to prevent the spread of disease, such as cleansing and disinfecting vehicles and equipment (16.1.1). It can be as simple as washing one's hands.

16.1.1 DEFRA's eight key precautions against FMD

1. Keep livestock separate
2. Deal with sheep last
3. Keep yourself clean
4. Keep the farm secure
5. Keep unnecessary vehicles away
6. Clean and disinfect
7. Avoid visiting other farms
8. Look for early signs of disease

Source: DEFRA

As biosecurity contributes greatly to disease prevention and control, it should be part of routine farming practice. The pig farming sector has already understood this. Most pig farmers learned the lesson from the classical swine fever outbreak in 2000 and increased their biosecurity standards.

However, in the FMD epidemic, the implementation of good biosecurity practice was patchy. The Trading Standards Institute commented that, *"…the concept of disinfection as well as cleaning with water was new to many in the farming community."* There were claims that vets and Government officials breached biosecurity. DEFRA informed us that they investigated all such claims. In most cases, they were shown to be groundless. However, it seems likely there were some breaches of tight biosecurity by officials and contractors. Although it can never be proved, this may have contributed to disease spread.

60. We recommend that farmers, vets and others involved in the livestock industry have access to training in biosecurity measures. Such training should form an integral part of courses at agricultural colleges.

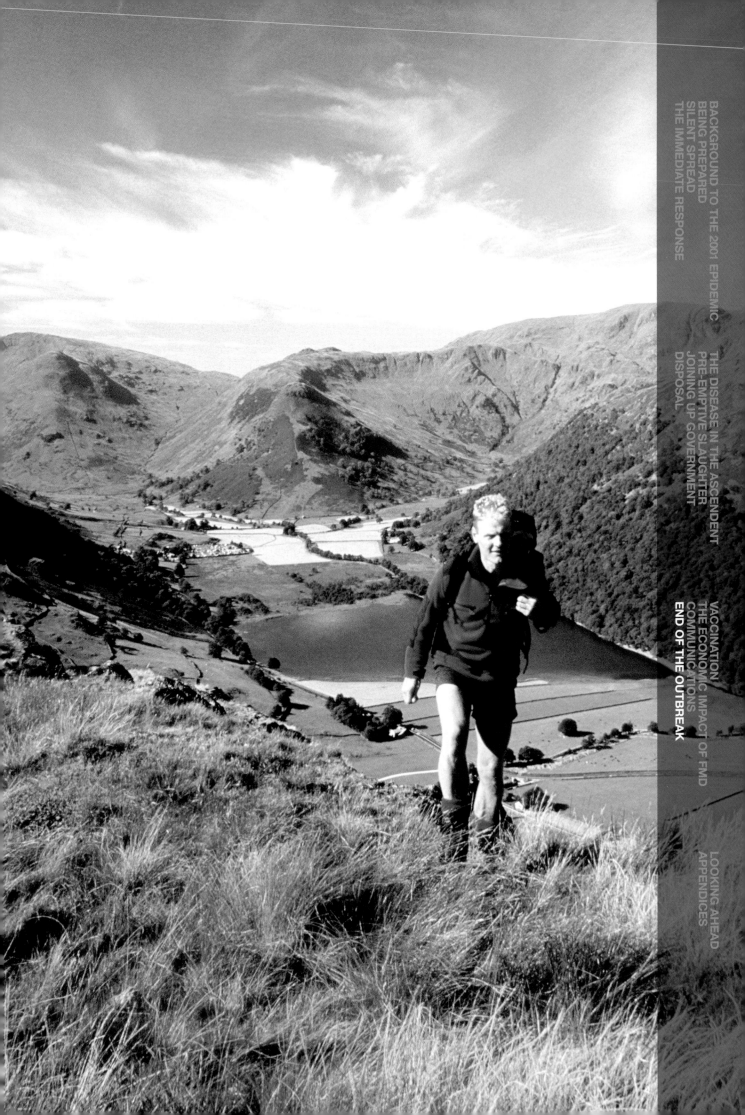

BACKGROUND TO THE 2001 EPIDEMIC
BEING PREPARED
SILENT SPREAD
THE IMMEDIATE RESPONSE

THE DISEASE IN THE ASCENDENT
PRE-EMPTIVE SLAUGHTER
JOINING UP GOVERNMENT
DISPOSAL

VACCINATION
THE ECONOMIC IMPACT OF FMD
COMMUNICATIONS
END OF THE OUTBREAK

LOOKING AHEAD
APPENDICES

"They [MAFF/DEFRA] would give us [Royal Welsh Showground, Builth Wells] permission to hold a Pony Club event here in the same week as they would not give us permission to have an Afghan hound show. When you asked them why they said we believe that horse owners will walk their horses over straw but we don't think that Afghan hound dog owners will walk their dogs over the same mats."

Public Meeting, regional visit to Wales

Understanding of biosecurity across the countryside was mixed. Disinfectant-soaked mats or straw that lay across roads raised public awareness, but many were of limited practical value. The disinfection area needed to be wide enough, regularly cleaned and replenished in order to do its job. Some mats were allowed to become filthy and to dry out. Others were too small.

61. **We recommend that the livestock industry and government jointly develop codes of practice on biosecurity. They should explore ways to communicate effectively with all practitioners and how incentives might be used to raise standards.**

At the start of the outbreak, MAFF prepared information on biosecurity, which was mailed and put on its website on 5 March. Several communications and reminders to farmers about biosecurity were made during the outbreak. Organisations such as the farmers' unions distributed information to their members. Limited resources prevented monitoring and enforcement of the procedures. Even though farmers realised these were important, some did not implement measures as rigorously or as often as they should. Some did not know what to do, and others found biosecurity difficult to implement and a burden to normal farming practice. Motivation to clean and disinfect a farm vehicle as it passed from location to location was low if the disease was not apparent. Washing soda is an effective disinfectant for FMD, but many bought expensive disinfectants unnecessarily.

On 10 May, FMD was reported in Settle. Sheep in the area had passed through Longtown market in February, but the disease did not become apparent until the cattle were let out onto pasture and became infected. Despite control measures employed at the time, the disease spread. Since infection could be traced to normal farming practices, such as movement of people or equipment between different locations, further attempts to improve levels of biosecurity were required. In June, a video was produced and, on 6 July, it was distributed to farmers. It emphasised the importance of biosecurity and outlined eight key precautions.

As the disease was dying out across most of the country, resources could be focused on 'hotspots' that sprang up in the late summer. The Thirsk cluster of cases caused alarm because the disease could have spread to the dense pig farming areas to the east. On 29 July, the first Restricted Infected Area, the so-called 'Blue Box', was declared and introduced strict enforcement of biosecurity and movement restrictions (16.1.2). Two more 'Blue Boxes' were declared – around the Penrith spur on 7 August and around Allendale and Hexham on 26 August.

16.1.2 Thirsk 'Blue Box'

A key aim of the Thirsk Restricted Infected Area or 'Blue Box', (so named because of the ink colour outlining the designated restricted area on the map), was to stop the spread of FMD between farms by either animal or human traffic. The enhanced biosecurity enforcement measures ran from 29 July to 14 September 2001. The roughly square 'Box' covered an area of North Yorkshire encompassing approximately 1,173 farms with susceptible livestock.

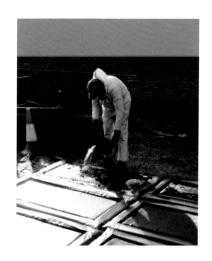

All vehicles visiting these farms required licences.

The enforcement effort was also backed by a major blood testing exercise to identify any residual pockets of the disease. There were no further outbreaks of the disease within the 'Box' after 18 August.

The whole operation, including planning, control, communications, use of intelligence and resulting enforcement action, was carried out by North Yorkshire County Council Trading Standards Service. The responsibility for enforcement of the Animal Health Act 1981 and its assorted legislation rests with the local authorities and, in the main, is delegated to the Trading Standards Service.

The restricted area was split into six sections, and trading standards and police carried out 15 patrols each day. The trading standards officers were accompanied at all times by the police who assisted by providing transport, stopping vehicles and by preventing breaches of the peace. The patrols carried out spot checks on more than 5,000 vehicles and 8,000 foot-baths. In addition, over 4,500 farm visits by milk tankers and feed lorries were supervised by DEFRA officials. Infringements at the end of the initiative were down to 5% from 15% at the start.

A total of 77 infringements were considered for legal action by trading standards officers. This threat of prosecution played a key role, in the view of the trading standards and veterinary staff involved, in stamping out the disease in the area at the same time as raising the profile and importance of biosecurity across the whole region.

Until the imposition of Restricted Infected Areas, biosecurity measures were not implemented effectively. Almost 80% of the spread of the disease was 'local' (16.1.3). This suggested breaches in biosecurity. Some argue that more emphasis on preventing spread by movement restrictions and biosecurity, in addition to rapid slaughter of infected premises and dangerous contacts would have been sufficient to control the epidemic without pre-emptive slaughter strategies.

62. We recommend that the use of Restricted Infected Area ('Blue Box' Biosecurity arrangements) procedures be built into contingency plans.

16.1.3 Methods of spread

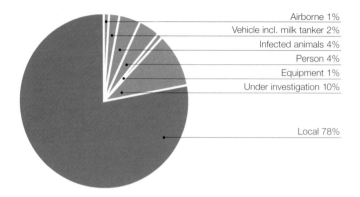

Airborne 1%
Vehicle incl. milk tanker 2%
Infected animals 4%
Person 4%
Equipment 1%
Under investigation 10%

Local 78%

Source: DEFRA (data at 21 October 2001)

When the most likely source of infection for each infected premises was traced, the majority of infected premises were due to 'local' spread. 'Local' here meant a new infected premise within 3km of another infected premise and where there was more than one means of spreading infection could be identified. The spread was likely to have been due to movements of people, vehicles or equipment, or spread between animals in close proximity.

(Of the 2,023 cases traced, suspect swill was implicated in only one instance, namely the index case at Burnside Farm, Heddon-on-the-Wall.)

16.2 Autumn movements

The seasonal pattern of the livestock industry necessitates extensive animal movements during the autumn. Without movements on this scale, serious welfare problems develop very quickly. Livestock movements, however, represent an epidemiological risk – which is why restrictions on movements are an important disease control measure. DEFRA and the industry knew that a tension would develop between these two opposing demands, and that it would need to be resolved by the autumn. This was the genesis of what would eventually become the Autumn Livestock Movement Scheme.

There were conflicting views within Government. On the one hand, the Chief Scientific Adviser was concerned that permitting extensive movements would undermine the seemingly fragile control that had been established over the disease, particularly in view of the fresh outbreaks in North Yorkshire and the North East in the summer. On the other, DEFRA and the Chief Veterinary Officer wished to ensure that the Scheme would go sufficiently far to meet the needs of the livestock industry that it would avoid widespread non-compliance.

Although both points of view were valid, they were not resolved until late in the development of Autumn Livestock Movement Scheme. As a result, finalisation of the policy was delayed by three to four weeks. It was not until 17 August that work began to develop the computer systems that would underpin the Scheme. With the Scheme due to become operational just one month later, on 17 September, the chances of a successful launch were low.

The delays impacted on the clarity with which the Scheme could be communicated to those affected and on the time available for local authorities, who would deliver the Scheme, to get their own computer systems up and running. Despite considerable effort on the part of the local authorities, it was an almost impossible task. During the first fortnight of September, the Local Authorities' Co-ordinating Body on Food and Trading Standards repeatedly pressed DEFRA to defer the start date.

From the outset, the computer system that supported the Scheme did not function as planned. There were problems of capacity and with the system's ability to approve or reject applications on the basis of geographic and disease control information.

As one local authority put it: *"We received in excess of 300 applications [on the first day of the Scheme] with a similar number received today. We were unable to access the DEFRA Autumn Livestock Movement Scheme computer until 1630 hours yesterday. When we did access the system we found the applications that we were submitting were refused in each case and this was despite a manual cross reference proving that the application should have been accepted. The computer system did not provide any meaningful or satisfactory reason for the refusal. Of course by the time we realised this was not just a one off problem, the DEFRA helpline to local authorities had closed."*

In addition, and in common with the Livestock Welfare (Disposal) Scheme, many staff who operated the Autumn Livestock Movement Scheme helplines had little initial knowledge of the Scheme. Later on, however, staff were allocated to manage relationships with individual farmers. The Scheme improved considerably as a result of this action.

For some farmers, the confusion surrounding the Autumn Livestock Movement Scheme was the final straw. A farming representative in the Tees Valley told us that, for hill farmers, it was the worst experience they had during the entire outbreak. Many were in desperation after months of restrictions.

In trying to strike the right balance between risk management and compliance, it would probably have been impossible to satisfy in full the requirements of the farming industry. However, their hopes and expectations of what the system would be capable of delivering turned to confusion, frustration and anger.

63. We recommend that disease control policies be developed in consultation with those local authorities responsible for implementing them.

The Scottish Executive did not need to manage autumn movements in the same way as DEFRA. Scotland was designated disease free on 11 September and was able to relax restrictions on animal movements. While Scotland was still fighting the disease, its policies had slight differences from those in England and Wales. However, from this point, policy development began to differ significantly.

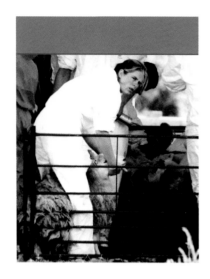

16.3.1 Serological surveillance

Serological surveillance provides statistical proof that FMD is no longer present in the country. Blood samples are tested for specific antibodies which will indicate if an animal has been infected with FMD. If the blood tests are negative, disease-free status can be regained after three months of the last FMD case, if vaccination is not used. If new cases are detected during the surveillance programme, the clock is set to zero.

The serological tests were similar to those used for diagnosis (8.1.1). During the outbreak, the Pirbright Laboratory validated the solid phase competitive (SPC) ELISA which allowed more samples to be tested than the original liquid phase blocking (LPB) ELISA. Inconclusive results were confirmed by the virus neutralisation test.

All the sheep that tested positive were killed. During the heat of the crisis, when the virus was actively circulating, positive sheep were confirmed as FMD cases. As the disease declined, veterinary judgement was applied to decide whether the result confirmed a case or not, especially when only one sheep in the flock tested positive. Further investigations, such as testing throat fluid samples for FMD virus, were conducted as necessary. If the sheep had recovered from the disease and virus was no longer present, FMD was not confirmed and the other animals were saved from slaughter.

16.3 Exit strategy

During the heat of the crisis, the priority had been disease eradication, with MAFF in 'fire fighting' mode. As the disease declined and officials perceived the end to be in sight, they were able to consider forward planning. Towards the end of April, they began to formulate the 'exit strategy'.

A crisis exit strategy is a plan for returning to normal. In the specific case of the FMD outbreak, several objectives influenced thinking: the need to demonstrate that the UK was free from FMD; the need to remove FMD restrictions around the country; the desirability of returning to EU and international trade; the need to resume normal domestic livestock trade; the aim of reopening the countryside and recovering domestic and international tourism. All of these were linked to regaining internationally recognised FMD-free status. The International animal health organisation, the OIE, set the standards for this, but, in practical terms, the EU's approval and requirements were paramount.

Different exit strategy approaches were assessed depending on the balance of priorities, and within the context of continued disease control. If the domestic situation was a priority, restrictions could be unwound, allowing the countryside and rural businesses, especially tourism, to return to normal as soon as areas were free of disease. By contrast, if international trade was a priority, restrictions would need to remain until the EU was satisfied that the areas were demonstrably free of disease via strict serological surveillance (16.3.1) within the 3km Protection Zones and 10km Surveillance Zones.

From May to July 2001, exit strategy options were negotiated with the EU. They were considered, with input from economic cost/benefit analyses and in consultation with industry representatives. Although regionalisation had been a possibility (Northern Ireland had earlier been recognised as FMD-free), Great Britain was treated on a whole country basis – England, Scotland and Wales – by the EU Standing Veterinary Committee and the OIE, as regards exports and disease freestatus. Restrictions on exports were gradually lifted county by county from October.

The exit strategy depended on the UK's serological testing capacity. Before the outbreak, the Pirbright Laboratory had been able to test about 400 ELISA samples a week. With increased resources, often due to the voluntary return of former staff or students, it was able, by April-May, to test 40,000 ELISA samples a week. From May onwards, other facilities were engaged to perform ELISA tests: Centre for Applied Microbiology and Research at Porton Down; various Veterinary Laboratories Agency facilities; and the Animal Health Trust at Newmarket. By the end of the outbreak, testing capacity was 200,000 ELISAs per week. Only the Pirbright Laboratory, however, had the appropriate containment facilities to conduct the confirmatory virus neutralisation tests.

The handling of the exit strategy would have been more straightforward and some issues not have arisen, if the Government had been better prepared in the early stages of the crisis.

16.4 UK declared FMD-free

The last confirmed case was in Appleby, Cumbria on 30 September 2001, 221 days after the first. However, not until three months after the last infected animal was slaughtered, with completion of the required surveillance, could the UK be declared disease free. All counties became FMD-free on 15 January 2002 and the UK regained its international FMD-free status at an OIE meeting on 22 January 2002. The EU Standing Veterinary Committee lifted the remaining export restrictions on 5 February 2002.

In looking ahead we return to our three principal aims set out in section 3 – keeping disease at bay, reducing vulnerability and minimising the impact of any future outbreaks.

The focus of our Inquiry was the 2001 FMD outbreak. But the lessons to be learned have wider applicability. The purpose of our recommendations is to help prepare the country for the range of exotic diseases which pose a potential threat. Disease control is an international issue. The UK contributes to global policy individually and through its membership of the European Union and the OIE. Our recommendations are designed to help the UK shape the framework of international regulations.

17.1 Keeping disease at bay

The OIE List A sets out those exotic diseases which can spread rapidly. An outbreak of any of these diseases can have severe economic consequences and implications for international trade (17.1.1).

The general tools for disease control are stamping out, movement restrictions, biosecurity and, if appropriate, vaccination. The control strategies for a given disease depend on its biological characteristics, on species susceptibility, on the methods of transmission, and on the availability and effectiveness of vaccines.

Swine vesicular disease only affects pigs. The clinical signs of swine vesicular disease and FMD in pigs are indistinguishable, but the implications of the diagnosis are significantly different. The OIE is considering the removal of swine vesicular disease from List A. But the consequences of a suspect case of FMD not being reported because it is dismissed as swine vesicular disease are serious.

64. We recommend that the UK should urge the OIE to consider the implications, for the detection and control of FMD, of the removal of swine vesicular disease from the List A of notifiable diseases.

Swine vesicular disease, classical swine fever and FMD can all be carried to the UK on the wind. For example, the small 1981 FMD outbreak on the Isle of Wight occurred when airborne virus was spread from Brittany. Such transmission can not be prevented although, as in 1981, there may be advance warning of the risk.

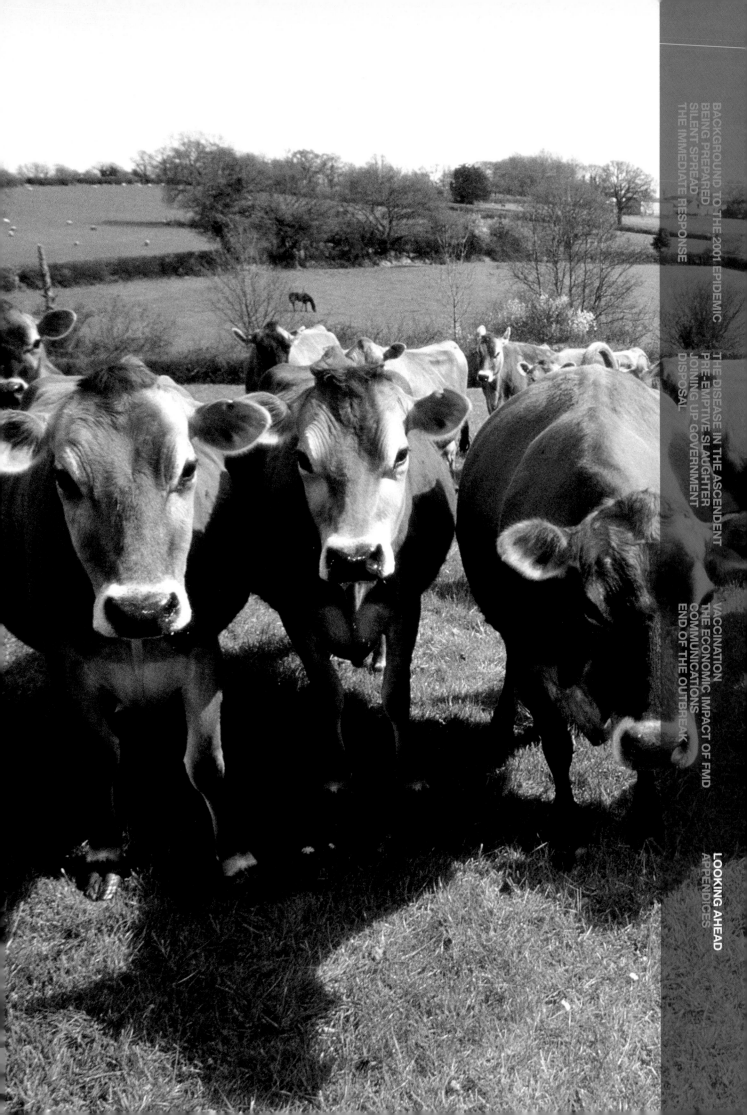

17.1.1 International Animal Health Code List A diseases

Foot and mouth disease	Bluetongue*
Vesicular stomatitis	Sheep pox and goat pox
Swine vesicular disease	African horse sickness*
Rinderpest	African swine fever*
Peste des petits ruminants	Classical swine fever*
Contagious bovine pleuropneumonia	Highly pathogenic avian influenza*
Lumpy skin disease	Newcastle disease*
Rift Valley fever	

Those marked * are discussed by the Royal Society in its Inquiry into Infectious Diseases in Livestock.

Illegal Imports Forum

Illegally imported, contaminated meat is another potential entry route.

DEFRA has an action plan to reduce the risk of exotic animal and plant disease entering the country. The key elements are:

- Risk assessment;
- Co-operation between agencies to achieve effective inter-agency co-ordination of checks;
- Effective intelligence to target smuggling;
- Legal powers to give enforcement officers new powers from April 2002 to search baggage, etc, for illegal imports of meat;
- European action to clarify and, if necessary, tighten enforcement of rules on third country imports reaching the UK via other EU states; to reform rules on personal imports;
- Publicity to clarify the UK's rules on imports of animal and plant products, and the reasons for them;
- Deterrence to give better information to passengers and shippers of the consequences of bringing illegal food imports into the UK.

To take this programme forward DEFRA held an 'Illegal Imports Forum' earlier this year. The farming unions in England, Scotland and Wales, representatives of Local Authorities, the Port Authorities, HM Customs and Excise, meat importers, airline companies and others attended the Forum.

Horizon scanning and surveillance

The risk of introduction of disease by illegal imports cannot be entirely eliminated. Horizon scanning – assessing the magnitude and location of global threats to pick up early warning signs is necessary. The role of the Civil Contingencies Secretariat in horizon scanning has been described in section 11.

The role of the Pirbright Laboratory

The Pirbright Laboratory plays a vital role in horizon scanning. As the World Reference Laboratory for FMD and seven other diseases classified as List A by the OIE, it holds data on reported outbreaks from around the world. In addition to research, the Pirbright Laboratory provides statutory diagnostic, surveillance and testing services to DEFRA, the Council of the European Commission, the OIE and the UN's Food and Agriculture Organisation. It also maintains a vaccination bank.

Under normal circumstances DEFRA funds projects at Pirbright on an annual basis. DEFRA's Science Directorate, the State Veterinary Service and the Biotechnology and Biological Sciences Research Council all fund strands of the Pirbright Laboratory's research and surveillance work. There is no coherent assessment of the full range of work undertaken by Pirbright in relation to the national surveillance and control strategies. In our view there should be.

The service arrangements in place in 2001, covered the processing of 300 samples a year for MAFF, but contained no procedure for increasing the level of provision in an emergency. The Pirbright Laboratory met the huge demand placed upon it during the outbreak as the result of extraordinary effort by those concerned, including a number of former staff and research students who volunteered to return to the laboratory to help.

Pirbright handled 15,500 diagnostic samples and over one million serology samples. It used additional laboratories, and brought in personnel from other establishments. But the contractual arrangements to support this activity were only put in place after the event.

The arrangements for funding, planning and monitoring the performance of the Pirbright Laboratory should be strengthened and formalised. Pirbright did not itself have in place a contingency plan for managing large-scale epidemics. The Laboratory was not consulted when the original FMD contingency plans were drawn up. The only reference to the Laboratory in DEFRA's current interim FMD contingency plan relates to training.

In recent years, Pirbright has experienced difficulties in recruiting and retaining staff at all levels. In 1983 it employed 13 vets. Now there are four.

65. **We recommend that the Pirbright Laboratory resources, and research programmes, be fully integrated into the national strategy for animal disease control, and budget provisions be made accordingly.**

Surveillance

A MAFF report on veterinary surveillance[1] in 1999-2000 commented on the *"major influence of expert advisory committees* [such as the Spongiform Encephalopathy Advisory Committee] *in determining surveillance priorities ... ... once recommendations are made by these committees they often become urgent political priorities for Government ... but because the recommendations of the committees are taken up on an ad hoc basis they can have major resource consequences... A clear published strategy for veterinary surveillance may assist in accommodating these external demands more efficiently."*

DEFRA is currently developing a strategy for enhancing UK veterinary surveillance of animal health.

66. **The State Veterinary Service, together with the Pirbright Laboratory, should increase their horizon scanning and threat assessment capabilities for major infectious animal diseases.**

Routine surveillance involves vets employed by the State Veterinary Service, the Meat Hygiene Service and the Veterinary Laboratories Agency, vets in private practice, and farmers and others working in the livestock industry. These agencies should all work closely together to achieve the common goals of the new surveillance strategy.

67. **We recommend that, in developing the surveillance strategy, there be the widest possible involvement of those with a role to play in surveillance.**

Veterinary recruitment

We have referred elsewhere to the difficulties in recruiting veterinary staff to the State Veterinary Service, especially in the South East, and to the reduced number of vets in large animal practice.

Demand for places on veterinary courses far exceeds availability. There may be scope in the longer term to increase the supply of places for veterinary training.

68. **We recommend that DEFRA and the Department for Education and Skills jointly explore with the veterinary professional bodies and higher education institutions the scope for increasing the capacity of undergraduate and postgraduate veterinary provision. Equivalent work should be done in Scotland and Wales.**

There were many occasions during the 2001 epidemic when vets in short supply were overburdened with animal health tasks that could have been done by someone with a lower level of expertise. There may be merit in recognising this and developing the concept of the veterinary 'paramedic'.

69. **We recommend that Government develop opportunities for increased use of veterinary 'paramedics'.**

The issue of recruitment and retention of State Veterinary Service vets dates back at least to the time of the 1968 Northumberland Report. The shortage

[1] Veterinary Surveillance in England and Wales: A review 1999/2000

of vets varies across the country. The most acute pressure on the State Veterinary Service is in London and the South East. By contrast, recruitment in Scotland and Wales is easier. The Chief Veterinary Officer told us that the State Veterinary Service had tried ways to address this, including salary increases, but with only limited success. Tackling recruitment and linking it to the availability of vets is sensible. Reducing the number of vets based in central London and increasing the number of posts in the regions would have the added advantage of increasing the level of veterinary expertise available in the regions to manage future disease outbreaks.

70. **We recommend that as many functions of the State Veterinary Service as possible be relocated from London, to regional centres, particularly to Scotland and Wales.**

17.2 Reducing vulnerability

The goal we have set out is one of gradual reduction of risk. Increasing knowledge and expertise in the industry will help to achieve that goal.

Agricultural education and training

Vets, farmers and others involved with the 2001 FMD epidemic told us that there were wide variations in the level of knowledge of animal diseases and how best to implement animal health and biosecurity practices. Farmers have an important part to play in monitoring animal health and in disease control. Yet training is minimal. For example, take-up of training within the agriculture industry is currently low, at 1.9 days per person per year on average.

Better biosecurity procedures are required. We have heard anecdotal reports that biosecurity standards have already started to slip since the end of the FMD outbreak.

Colleges, universities and training organisations should ensure therefore that their curriculum reflects changing demands on those working in the livestock industry. Additional support should be provided to increase understanding of the importance of biosecurity.

71. **We recommend that Government support a national action group charged with the responsibility of producing a plan to tackle the gaps in practitioners' knowledge of preventing and managing infectious diseases of livestock. To be effective this will need a timetable, milestones for achievement and incentives.**

72. **We recommend that colleges, universities and training organisations provide courses to equip those working in the food and livestock industries, and those owning susceptible animals, with the skills and knowledge to enable them to recognise the signs of animal disease early and take appropriate action to prevent its spread.**

The report of the Policy Commission on the Future of Farming and Food made a number of recommendations on developing knowledge and skills, which we endorse.

The Government announced on 26 March 2002 its intention to 'carry out a review of the effectiveness of training and education provision for farmers and other land managers'.

The experience gained by the farmers, vets and others who experienced the 2001 outbreak must be captured and kept alive.

73. **We recommend that DEFRA commission a handbook for farmers on identifying and responding to animal disease, drawing on the experience of 2001.**

It is essential that the high level of knowledge and expertise about FMD that has been generated during the 2001 epidemic is not lost but maintained for future generations to use.

74. **We recommend that training for Local Veterinary Inspectors in exotic diseases be intensified, and consolidated into ongoing training strategies.**

Farm assurance and licensing

The production of animal feedstuffs, the movement of livestock to slaughter and the slaughter process itself are all subject to regulation. Intensive pig and poultry farms are highly regulated.

By contrast, the day-to-day practices of the sheep farming sector are less tightly controlled.

The NFU told us that the agricultural industry has a permanent responsibility to maintain and improve standards of hygiene and biosecurity. The NFU believes that initiatives already in hand, such as the farm assurance schemes, are the best way to demonstrate quality and raise standards.

The report of the Policy Commission on the Future of Farming and Food discusses assurance schemes in some detail and makes related recommendations, which we endorse. Those recommendations do not, however, explicitly incorporate disease awareness and biosecurity.

75. **We recommend that farm assurance schemes take account of animal health and welfare, biosecurity, food safety and environmental issues.**

Further consideration should be given to more formal licensing systems. In particular, there is scope for examining whether so-called 'negative licensing' might provide further incentives. Under such arrangements, farmers and dealers would be issued with a licence which could be withdrawn following repeated infringements of codes of practice or failure to meet standards.

76. **We recommend that the livestock industry work with Government to undertake a thorough review of the assurance and licensing options to identify those arrangements most likely to reward good practice and take-up of training, and how such a new system might be implemented.**

17.3 Minimising the impact

Disease control strategies and the legal position

The Animal Health Act 1981 provides the legal basis for activities carried out by the Government to control animal diseases, including FMD. Schedule 3 of the Act relates to slaughter of animals to control FMD. It reads:

> SCH.3 *Foot-and-mouth disease*
>
> 3.–(1) The Minister may, if he thinks fit, in any case cause to be slaughtered–
>
> (a) any animals affected with foot-and-mouth disease, or suspected of being so affected; and
>
> (b) any animals which are or have been the same field, shed, or other place, on in the same herd or flock, or otherwise in contact with animals affected with foot-and-mouth disease, or which appear to the Minister to have been in any way exposed to the infection of foot-and-mouth disease.

The Act provides a legal basis for the slaughter of animals at infected premises, as well as animals classified as dangerous contacts. But the Act does not provide such a clear basis for control methods based on slaughtering animals where there are not grounds for suspecting that they have been exposed to infection.

Lord Whitty told the Inquiry that the legality of the contiguous cull had been "an issue". The Act permits slaughter of animals 'which appear to the Minister to have been in any way exposed to the infection of foot-and-mouth disease'. The Minister, acting on the advice of his senior veterinary advisers, judged animals on contiguous premises to have been exposed to FMD. Those premises were, therefore, culled on that assumption.

It is a matter for the courts to determine whether the powers available to the Minister were sufficient to support the use of the contiguous cull as a disease control strategy. However, we consider the powers to be insufficiently clear. This lack of clarity contributed to a sense of mistrust of the Government, which was made worse by poor communication of the rationale of the cull.

77. **We recommend that the powers available in the Animal Health Act 1981 be re-examined, possibly in the context of a wider review of animal health legislation, to remove any ambiguity over the legal basis for future disease control strategies.**

Restrictions on animal movements

The intermingling of animals that occurred when sheep were bought and sold in markets in February 2001 was such a significant factor in transmitting infection that restrictions on movements after market exposure are still in place as a precaution against future spread of the disease. We listened to the arguments on the merits and practicalities of continuing to impose movement restrictions. We understand the economic and practical implications that such bans have for current farming practice.

But the consequences of relaxing these restrictions could, in some circumstances, be devastating. A long-term solution to the problem of movement restrictions must strike an appropriate balance between the legitimate interests of the industry and the need for long term disease control.

78. **We recommend that the Government retain the 20-day movement restrictions pending a detailed risk assessment and wide ranging cost-benefit analysis.**

This recommendation should be kept under review so that, should the risks change, a modified approach can be adopted.

Animal tracing and electronic tagging

Tracing of animal movements from Longtown Market was essential to the disease control effort. However, in the absence of a robust system for identifying the movements of individual sheep, MAFF had to appeal, as late as 8 March 2001, to farmers to come forward if they *"...believe they have received sheep from Longtown Market held on either 15 or 22 February..."*.

In future, animal identification should be by electronic tagging using the best available technology. There are practical implications of introducing such a policy that need to be worked out in detail, in advance. A full cost benefit analysis should be completed before the new system is introduced. There are many benefits, in terms of disease control, from such improved traceability.

The NFU, in its submission to the Inquiry, said that *"Cost-effective electronic identification and traceability of sheep must be developed and delivered to the industry as a matter of urgency."* The National Sheep Association told us that it would support *"the urgent development, funded by government, of electronic tagging of sheep to be deployed at an individual level if the technology was both reliable and affordable."* Trials both in Great Britain and abroad are already providing an encouraging foundation for progress.

79. **We recommend that Government develop a comprehensive livestock tracing system using electronic tags to cover cattle, sheep and pigs, taking account of developments at EU level. The Government should seek to lead the debate in Europe on this issue.**

Insurance and compensation

Much of the cost of the 2001 outbreak to the farming industry was externalised. Farmers whose animals were culled were entitled to compensatory payments under current legislation. The notion of value is particularly complex in large-scale outbreaks where the normal operation of the market may break down for long periods. The Northumberland Report discussed many of the issues surrounding valuation and made proposals for an indexed scheme to allow for valuation and immediate payment based on pre-outbreak prices and subsequent indexing to adjust compensation in the light of exit values.

Whether compensation is the appropriate reimbursement mechanism or whether a system closer to insurance arrangement should operate is a complex question. It is beyond the competence of this inquiry to judge the relative merits of compensation or insurance schemes, or to make recommendations about how such schemes might work.

DEFRA has set up the Working Group for Animal Disease Insurance, involving representatives of the farming and insurance industry. It provides a suitable forum for making progress in this area, and is putting proposals to Ministers.

Previous reports into FMD outbreaks concluded that compensation for consequential loss – whether for farmers who suffered losses because of movement restrictions, for rural tourist businesses who lost income through loss of customers, or for secondary industries affected by the loss of business in farming and tourism – is neither desirable nor feasible. We agree with this conclusion. The DEFRA working group is the appropriate forum to explore these matters further.

However, it is important to recognise the long-lasting divisions caused in rural communities by the perceived unfairness of providing compensation for only one small group of those affected. These effects should be taken fully into account during any consideration of compensation issues.

80. We recommend that the joint DEFRA Industry Working Group for Animal Disease Insurance ensure that its scope and membership is set widely enough to address valuation and compensation issues highlighted by the 2001 outbreak. Clear deadlines should be set for reporting progress.

Interim contingency plan

In March 2002, DEFRA published an interim FMD contingency plan to respond to deficiencies in the previous plan. It builds on the experience gained during the 2001 outbreak, particularly in the areas of initial response and command and control structures. A contingency plan for the use of vaccination as a disease control measure is being taken forward separately.

The interim plan has a number of gaps which may be filled by a process of consultation and the widest possible involvement of all the relevant stakeholders. We also expect the lessons identified by this and other inquiries be fully incorporated in the final document.

81. We recommend that DEFRA develop further its interim plan, published in March 2002, in full consultation with all interested parties. Its relevance should be maintained through agreed programmes of rehearsal, practice, review and reporting. This work should be given priority for funding.

FOOT
AND
MOUTH
DISEASE
2001:
LESSONS
TO BE
LEARNED
INQUIRY
APPENDICES

18.1 Glossary of terms

FMD terms and definitions	
Antibody	Specialised proteins in the blood that are produced as part of an immune response to foreign material.
Biosecurity	Precautions taken to minimise the risk that the virus might be spread inadvertently by those working with livestock and visiting farms, and after infected animals have been slaughtered and disposed of. These include thorough cleansing and disinfecting of premises where animals that had been infected or exposed were present.
'Blue Box' (Restricted Infected Area)	An area where very strict biosecurity measures are imposed, including biosecurity of vehicles around a designated area and a ban on almost all animal movements, except for those direct to slaughter.
Case	An occurrence of FMD on a particular premises where one or more animal in a flock or herd is affected with the disease.
'Clean' Vet	A vet who has not been exposed to infection or who, having been exposed or potentially exposed to infection, has carried out personal cleansing and disinfection and has completed the required quarantine period.
Clinical	The observation and treatment of actual patients rather than laboratory studies. When used to describe a disease or condition, the term means causing observable and recognisable symptoms.
Contiguous premises	A category of dangerous contacts where animals may have been exposed to infection on neighbouring infected premises.
Controlled Area	The area affected by general control on movement of susceptible animals.
Dangerous contacts	Premises where animals have been in direct contact with infected animals or have, in any way, been exposed to infection.
'Dirty' vet	A vet who has been exposed or potentially exposed to infection and who has not completed the required quarantine period.
Drover	A person who herds cattle or sheep to market or pasture.
ELISA (Enzyme-linked immunosorbent assay)	Laboratory test using antibodies to detect the material of interest.
Endemic	An endemic disease is one present in an animal population at all times.
Epidemic	A disease affecting, or tending to affect, a disproportionately large number of individuals within a population, community or region at the same time.
Epizootic	A disease which affects a large number of animals in a large area at the same time and spreads rapidly. The equivalent term to epidemic in humans.
Epidemiology	The statistical study of populations, and the patterns of diseases from which they suffer, with the aim of determining the events or circumstances causing these diseases and their spread.
Form A	A notice of suspected disease on premises from the start of a report case either until it is declared negative, or until, after confirmation, cleansing and disinfection and any restocking procedures have been completed.
Form D	A notice imposing restrictions on an owner or person in charge of animals exposed to infection or to an occupier of premises where such animals are situated. It is served where the intention is to observe animals rather than slaughter them as dangerous contacts. The restrictions include that no person shall permit any animal to move or be moved in or out of the premises except under licence and that no animal product may be moved in or out of the premises. Cleansing and disinfection measures must be in force.

FMD terms and definitions continued

Hogget	A yearling sheep, between weaning and first shearing.
Incubation period	The incubation period of a disease is the time from when an animal first becomes infected to when it first exhibits clinical signs of disease. The incubation period is dependent on the dose of the virus, the route of transmission, the strain of the virus, the animal species and the conditions under which they are kept.
Infected animal	An infected animal is an animal which receives a sufficient dose of FMD virus such that it will go on to replicate the virus, excrete it and develop clinical disease.
Infected Areas	Areas under Infected Area Order Restrictions. On confirmation of FMD an Infected Area is imposed which extends to a minimum of 10km around the infected place.
Infected premises	Premises where FMD has been confirmed on clinical grounds by a vet or by a positive result in a laboratory test. Cases for which the subsequent laboratory tests prove negative are still counted as infected premises because a negative test does not necessarily mean that the animal was not infected
Index case	The source case to which all other cases can be traced back, in a specified outbreak of disease or infection, in a particular region.
InterSpread	The epidemiological model used by the Veterinary Laboratories Agency.
Lesion	A blister, ulcer or abscess
Light lamb	A light lamb, under the 2001 Livestock Welfare (Disposal) Scheme, was defined as one born since January 2001.
Livestock Welfare (Disposal) Scheme	A scheme for farmers whose livestock were facing welfare problems as a result of the movement restrictions related to FMD.
'Page Street'	Location of MAFF/DEFRA Departmental Emergency Control Centre and Joint Co-ordination Centre, based in 1A Page Street, London SW1.
Protection zone	The area within a 3km boundary of an Infected Premises. Form D restrictions applied within the zone.
Rendering	The process involving the crushing of internal organs, entrails and other parts of discarded animal carcasses, followed by the indirect application of heat, enabling the separation of the 'tallow' (fat) and the 'greaves' (high protein solids), which are further processed to make meat and bone meal.
Serology	The scientific study of blood serum and antibodies.
Slaughter on suspicion	Premises where a veterinary inspection detects symptoms of the disease, but which were insufficient to confirm that FMD is present, and where animals were culled. If subsequent tests confirmed the disease the premises were classified as infected premises; cases which have proven negative or remain unconfirmed remain classified as slaughter on suspicion.
Swill	Food waste mixed with water for feeding to pigs.

18.2 Key facts

Some of the statistics showing the scale and impact of the epidemic are disputed. Different organisations have published statistics about the events. Some data are still being finalised. As discussed, in sections 9.3 and 11.3, there were no consistent and rigorous systems in place to collect the data and ensure their accuracy, especially in the early days of the crisis. While data collection understandably took second place to disease control for those on the ground, everyone directing the strategy from the centre needed accurate and up-to-date information to gauge how effectively policies were working and how they needed to change.

The following are some of the key facts and figures which illustrate the nature of the crisis.

There were 2,026 cases, or infected premises, in mainland Great Britain. The total for the UK as whole, including the four cases in Northern Ireland, is 2,030. Pre-emptive culling was carried out on a further 8,131 premises.

18.2.1 Numbers of cases confirmed per week, and total

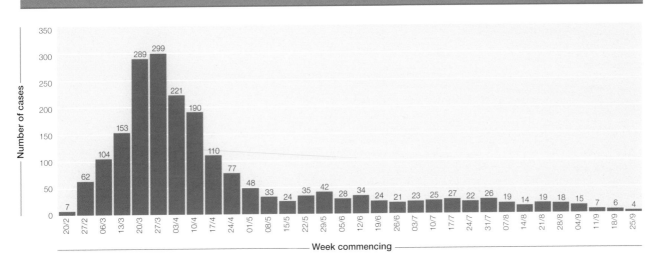

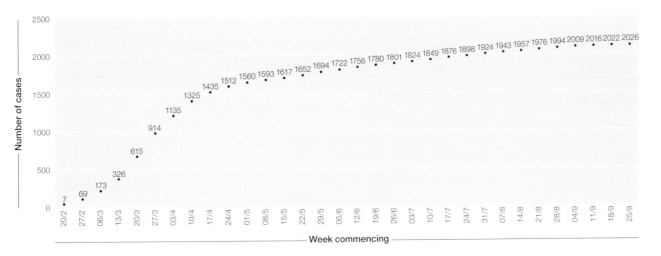

18.2.2 Total numbers of infected premises, dangerous contacts, and contiguous premises

Infected premises	Dangerous contacts	Contiguous premises	Total
2,026	4,762	3,369	10,157

Source: DEFRA

Figures for infected premises (18.2.2) include some cases where subsequent laboratory tests proved negative, although this does not mean necessarily that the animal was not infected. Slaughter on suspicion cases giving positive results or subsequently confirmed on clinical grounds, are classified as infected premises.

Animals slaughtered as part of a 3km cull were recorded as dangerous contacts, not contiguous premises, and will therefore include animals on some premises in Scotland, Wales and Cumbria that would otherwise have been regarded as contiguous.

18.2.3 Number of animals slaughtered for disease control and welfare purposes

	Disease control				Welfare
	Infected premises	Dangerous contact contiguous premises	Dangerous contact non-contiguous premises (including 3km cull)	Slaughter on suspicion	
Sheep	968,000	991,000	1,360,000	109,000	1,821,000
Cattle	301,000	196,000	82,000	13,000	166,000
Pigs	22,000	50,000	68,000	3,000	306,000
Total					6,456,000

Source: National Audit Office

The figures above (18.2.3) exclude around 4,000 other animals, chiefly goats and deer, slaughtered for disease control purposes, and around 3,000 other animals slaughtered under the Livestock Welfare (Disposal) Scheme.

They also exclude a large number of new born lambs and calves not counted by MAFF/DEFRA's database because, for the purposes of valuing, they were counted with their mother. It has not been possible accurately to estimate the number of lambs and calves involved. The total of 6.5 million animals slaughtered is, therefore, lower than some other estimates. (For example, articles in the press claimed that over ten million animals were slaughtered. This figure, which was wrongly attributed to the Meat and Livestock Commission, would allow for the slaughter of an additional 1.2 million lambs killed with breeding sheep.)

The totals slaughtered for welfare reasons included 1,768,000 sheep, cattle and pigs slaughtered under the Livestock Welfare (Disposal) Scheme, and 525,000 lambs under the Light Lambs Scheme. The purpose of the Light Lambs Scheme, which ran between 3 September and 26 October 2001, was to slaughter those lambs which faced welfare problems because of movement restrictions and the export ban.

18.2.4 Number of animals slaughtered for food

Number of animals slaughtered for human consumption

	End February – End September 2000	End February – End September 2001
Cattle	1,400,000	1,200,000
Sheep	9,900,000	6,500,000
Pigs	7,300,000	6,000,000

Source: DEFRA

18.2.5 Main disposal methods used during the outbreak

	Burning (including incineration, on-farm burning and mass pyres)	Rendering	Landfill (including mass burial)	Burying	Other
Pigs	39%	32%	18%	11%	2%
Cattle	41%	35%	16%	6%	1%
Sheep	27%	27%	24%	20%	2%
All	29%	28%	22%	18%	2%

Source: National Audit Office

Notes
Numbers have been rounded, so may not total 100. These figures do not include animals slaughtered under the Livestock Welfare (Disposal) Scheme or the 3km cull. The **other** category comprises animals disposed of in abattoirs, and those recorded as 'method uncertain, to be investigated further'.

18.3 Disease control statistics

Disease control statistics by local Disease Control Centre

Disease Control Centre	Affected Counties, Metropolitan Districts and Unitary Authorities covered	Number of confirmed cases (infected premises)[1]	Date of first confirmed case	Date of last confirmed case
Carlisle	Cumbria	891	28-Feb-01	30-Sep-01
Newcastle	Darlington; Durham; Newcastle-upon-Tyne; Northumberland; Stockton-on-Tees	190	23-Feb-01	29-Sep-01
Ayr and Dumfries	Dumfries and Galloway	177	01-Mar-01	23-May-01
Exeter	Devon	172	25-Feb-01	17-Jun-01
Leeds	Bradford; Leeds; North Yorkshire	140	07-Mar-01	18-Aug-01
Cardiff and Llandrindod Wells	Caerphilly; Monmouthshire; Newport; Neath Port Talbot; Powys; Rhondda, Cynon, Taff	101	28-Feb-01	12-Aug-01
Gloucester	Bristol; Gloucestershire; South Gloucestershire; Wiltshire	85	26-Feb-01	17-Apr-01
Worcester	Herefordshire; Shropshire; Telford and Wrekin; Worcestershire,	79	27-Feb-01	11-May-01
Stafford	Cheshire; Derbyshire; Staffordshire	72	02-Mar-01	26-Jul-01
Preston	Lancashire; Warrington; Wigan	55	27-Feb-01	17-Jul-01
Caernarfon	Isle of Anglesey	13	27-Feb-01	24-Mar-01
Galashiels	Scottish Borders	11	28-Mar-01	30-May-01
Chelmsford	Essex; Greater London; Thurrock	11	20-Feb-01	12-Apr-01
Taunton	Somerset	9	08-Mar-01	17-Jun-01
Leicester	Leicestershire; Northamptonshire; Warwickshire	9	27-Feb-01	23-Apr-01
Reigate	Kent; Medway	5	10-Mar-01	02-Apr-01
Truro	Cornwall	4	02-Mar-01	06-Apr-01
Reading	Oxfordshire	2	03-Mar-01	15-Mar-01

Source: National Audit Office

Notes

[1] For certain local authority areas and counties, such as Cumbria, Devon and Dumfries and Galloway, there are small apparent differences between the number of infected premises shown here. This is because, in a few cases, where an infected premises lay on the edge of a county the case was sometimes handled by a Disease Control Centre in a neighbouring county.

Disease control statistics by local Disease Control Centre continued

Days with the disease	Number of vets working on 10 April 2001[2]	% of confirmed cases which tested positive for the virus[3]	% of infected premises slaughtered out within 24 hours of report[3]	% of infected premises where disposal completed within 24 hours of slaughter[3]	Average number of dangerous contact premises for each infected premises	% of dangerous contact premises slaughtered out within 48 hours[3]
214	243	89	33	38	3	53
218	71	74	20	53	3	27
83	61	65	27	51	7	9
112	332	69	26	9	5	12
164	28	93	57	77	5	38
165	38	59	37	65	4	24
50	66	31	33	41	3	15
73	39	36	38	8	5	5
146	51	47	45	57	2	3
140	35	85	39	92	4	24
25	24	45	27	17	17	0
63	29	82	38	91	6	26
51	16	91	10	30	1	0
101	8	89	60	89	5	24
55	19	71	13	25	4	0
23	13	40	0	0	4	0
35	24	50	0	0	6	50
12	4	100	0	50	2	0

2 There were a further 51 state vets based at Animal Health Divisional Offices that did not have confirmed cases.

3 Based on analysis by DEFRA of data extracted from the Disease Control System in May 2002.
The figures are for the period of the entire epidemic.

18.4 Comparison with 1967-68

Between 1954 and 1967, isolated outbreaks of FMD in the UK had occurred almost every year. Consequently, at the time of the last major outbreak in 1967-68, there was much greater awareness of the disease. Some of the key differences between the 1967-68 and 2001 epidemics are shown in the following table:

	1967-68 epidemic	2001 epidemic
Date the first case was confirmed	25 October 1967, at Bryn Farm in Shropshire.	20 February 2001, at an abattoir in Essex.
Date the last case was diagnosed	4 June 1968.	30 September 2001.
Length of epidemic	222 days.	221 days.
Speed of identification of the source case	Reported to the Department's vet within four days of the onset of clinical signs.	Reported to the Department's vets around three weeks after the likely onset of clinical signs.
Extent of initial 'seeding'	There were up to 24 almost simultaneous primary outbreaks deriving from a consignment of infected frozen lamb carcasses from Argentina distributed in Cheshire and Shropshire. This led to an early explosion in cases, with 490 cases occurring during one week in mid-November 1967.	There was one source case, but its identification, three weeks after infection, meant the disease had been spread around the country as a result of movements of, mainly, sheep through markets and dealers. At least 57 premises, in nine geographical groups, are now known to have been 'seeded' with infection by 20 February 2001. Each case would be likely to give rise to further cases because of the infectious nature of the virus with the result that the outbreak would be extremely large.
The extent to which the disease spread throughout the UK (18.4.1)	The disease was mainly concentrated in the Cheshire Plain, affecting in particular dairying areas of Cheshire, Staffordshire, Montgomeryshire, Denbighshire, Shropshire and Flintshire. There were outbreaks in 16 counties.	The disease was widespread and affected 44 British counties, unitary authorities and metropolitan districts from the Scottish Borders in the north, to Anglesey in the west, and to Cornwall in the far south west. There were concentrations of infection in Cumbria, Devon, Dumfries and Galloway, Northumberland and North Yorkshire.
Overall number of infected premises (18.4.2)	2,364 The peak of the epidemic was higher and earlier than in 2001 because of the large number of simultaneous primary outbreaks.	2,026
Number of animals slaughtered for disease control purposes	442,000 (49% cattle, 26% pigs and 25% sheep).	More than four million (85% sheep, 12% cattle, 3% pigs).
Suspected source of infection	Infected frozen lamb imported from Argentina.	Infected imported animal products.
Cause of spread	Mainly airborne, with relative humidity and wind speed and direction assisting spread. Cattle were the main species affected by disease. From mid-February 1968 there were 18 cases of re-infection on farms which had restocked. In 12 of these, recrudescence arose from incomplete cleansing and disinfecting of farms.	Initially, by movements of infected animals, particularly sheep, in which the virus was present but clinical signs had not been detected. Later by local spread, including through persons, machinery and vehicles that had been in contact with infected animals and where compliance with biosecurity measures had not been effective.

Source: National Audit Office

Comparison with 1967-68 outbreak continued

	1967-68 epidemic	2001 epidemic
Cost to DEFRA	Around £370 million at 2001 prices, including £280 million paid out to farmers in compensation.	Over £3 billion, including £1.2 billion paid to farmers in compensation.
Introduction of national movement ban	After around a week, movement restrictions were extended to the counties adjacent to the Infected Areas to form a barrier zone and on 18 November 1967, 24 days into the epidemic, a Controlled Area (including national movement restrictions) was imposed across England and Wales. On 25 November, it was extended to Scotland.	A national movement ban was introduced just under three days after the first case had been officially confirmed.
State of UK livestock industry	Smaller and more compact farms. Fewer animal movements. Beef and sheep production more extensive, with the average number of livestock per holding less than half that in 2001. Movement of animals highly seasonal. Far fewer animals and much smaller land mass affected than in 2001.	Farm sizes and stock numbers have increased significantly since 1967-68, production cycles are shorter and seasonality has lessened. The livestock industry is more intensive and there are many more animal movements, particularly of sheep. As a result, the land mass of Great Britain affected and numbers of animals involved was considerably greater than in 1967-68, even though the number of cases was similar. While the cattle population had decreased by a quarter over the last 30 years to 9.5 million in Great Britain and the pig population by a half, to six million, the sheep population had grown by a half to 40 million in 2000, including 21 million breeding ewes. The sheep flock is the largest in the European Union.
Number of live auction markets in the UK	Over 800	170
Number of slaughterhouses in the UK	Over 3,000	Fewer than 500
Numbers of veterinary surgeons	An additional 645 vets were mobilised.	Over 1,800 vets were deployed at the peak of the outbreak.
Number of days before military deployed	12	25, though the Department had been liaising with the military from day 1.
Number of troops deployed	400	More than 2,000 at the peak.

18.4.1 Areas infected, 1967-68 and 2001

Infected premises by county – 1967-68 outbreak

Infected premises by county – 2001 outbreak

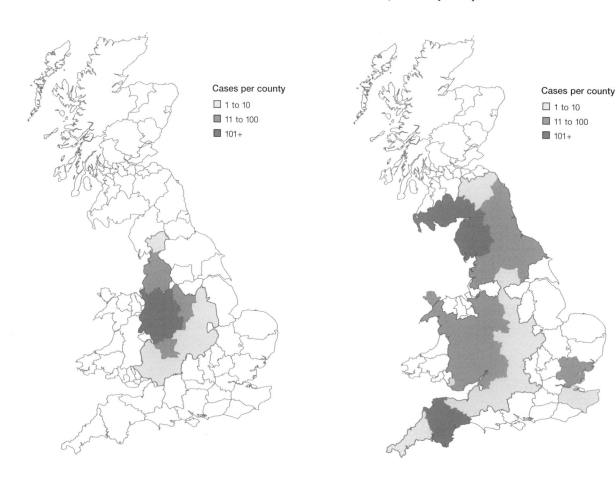

Cases per county
- ☐ 1 to 10
- ▨ 11 to 100
- ■ 101+

Cases per county
- ☐ 1 to 10
- ▨ 11 to 100
- ■ 101+

18.4.2 Comparison of number of cases confirmed per week, 1967-68 and 2001

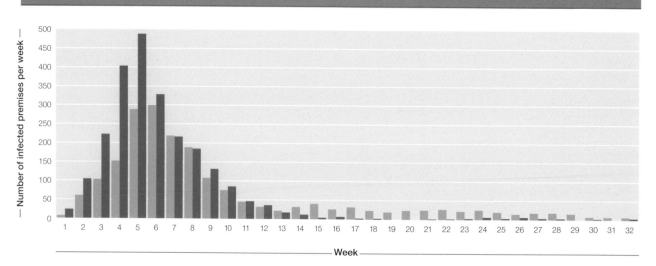

■ 1967-68   ▨ 2001

18.5 Scotland

The outbreak in Scotland	
Context 1. Size and importance of the livestock sector	Pre-outbreak: 9.2 million sheep, 2 million cattle, and 0.6 million pigs. Agriculture contributed 1.4% of Scotland's gross domestic product in 2000, with the livestock sector's share 52%.
Preparedness 2. Date local contingency plans last updated before the outbreak	Inverurie Animal Health Divisional Office in June 2000; Inverness in September 2000; Perth in January 2001; Ayr in February 2000; and Galashiels in August 2000.
3. Date of last simulation exercise	Local contingency plans were tested biennially by Animal Health Divisional Offices. The last exercise was held in Ayr in 1999.
4. Involvement of stakeholders	Local exercises involved local and headquarters' State Veterinary Service staff, Scottish Executive agricultural staff, local police, local authorities and Scottish Environment Protection Agency staff.
Course and extent of the outbreak 5. Date of confirmation of first case	1 March 2001, near Lockerbie in Dumfriesshire (reported by owner on 28 February 2001).
6. Date of confirmation of last case	30 May 2001 in Berwickshire.
7. Duration of outbreak between first and last cases	90 days. The peak of the epidemic was between 21 and 28 March 2001, when up to seven new cases were being reported daily.
8. Date declared free of the disease	11 September 2001.
9. Epidemiological groups and seeding	Two-main groups: Dumfries and Galloway, with 177 infected premises; and the Scottish Borders, with 11 cases. The Dumfries and Galloway cases were a subset of the larger Cumbria cluster. Disease was seeded by movements of animals and persons to and from Longtown Market, Cumbria, prior to 23 February 2001. The Scottish Borders' cases were a subset of the Northumberland epidemiological group.
10. Number of infected premises	187
11. Number of dangerous contact premises slaughtered-out	1,445[1]
12. Number of animals slaughtered on infected premises	132,000 – 73% sheep and 27% cattle[1].
13. Number of animals slaughtered on dangerous contact and slaughter on suspicion premises	624,000 – 90% sheep, 9% cattle and 1% pigs. 77% of these animals were slaughtered on premises non-contiguous to infected premises and 20% on contiguous premises, and 3% were 'slaughter on suspicion' cases.
14. Number of animals slaughtered for welfare reasons	307,000, including 188,000 'light lambs', 49,000 sheep, 59,000 pigs and 11,000 cattle.
15. Proportion of country under Infected Area restrictions at one time	10%, concentrated in the south, with two-thirds of farms in Dumfries and Galloway being affected.

Source: National Audit Office

Notes

[1] Data on animals slaughtered and numbers of infected premises are based on DEFRA's information. There are some small differences compared with the figures that have been presented by the Scottish Executive.

The outbreak in Scotland continued

Handling the outbreak

16. Animal Health arrangements

Under the Scotland Act of 1998, legislation on all animal health matters has been devolved to the Scottish Parliament and policy development and implementation made the responsibility of Scottish Ministers. However, the State Veterinary Service, headed by the Chief Veterinary Officer, has been retained as a Britain-wide body. This was because it was recognised that animal diseases show no respect for constitutional or geographical boundaries and there would be advantages from sharing research, analytical and veterinary resources. Concordats between the Scottish Executive and DEFRA set out an agreed framework for co-operation. They specify that DEFRA pays the compensation for notifiable diseases such as foot and mouth, but that the Scottish Executive provides the administrative support staff in State Veterinary Service offices in Scotland.

The Assistant Chief Veterinary Officer advises the Scottish Executive on animal health issues. The Scottish Executive's Environment and Rural Affairs Department advises Scottish Executive ministers on policy and implementation of policy.

During the 2001 outbreak, Scottish Ministers were responsible for policy, but were party to Great Britain decisions taken on its handling and the scientific advice on which it was based. They operated within an agreed policy framework while taking account of local disease circumstances, Scottish topography and farming practices and the views of stakeholders. Consequently, there were some variations in the detailed implementation of Great Britain policy, for example in the movement licensing regime.

17. Organisational structure during the 2001 outbreak

On 28 February 2001, a Disease Control Centre was set up at the Ayr Animal Health Divisional Office. The Divisional Veterinary Manager led on dealing with infected premises, dangerous contacts, epidemiology and surveillance. A Forward Field Station was also set up in Dumfries, close to the focus of infection using existing offices and the Dumfries and Galloway Council Emergency Centre. It included representatives from the emergency services, local authorities and the main contractor, Barr Limited.

On 26 March 2001, a tripartite Disease Strategy Group was set up in Edinburgh to have overall responsibility for management of the outbreak in Scotland. It comprised senior representatives from the Scottish Executive's Environment and Rural Affairs Department, the State Veterinary Service and the armed services and oversaw the strategy and resource allocation. It met twice daily, formalising the arrangements for daily meetings which had been in place since the start of the outbreak.

On 30 March 2001, two days after the first case of disease was confirmed in the Scottish Borders, a Command and Control Centre was set up at Galashiels Animal Health Division Office.

18. Regional Operations Director: date of appointment and role

20 March 2001.

Termed the 'Operations Co-ordinator', he was appointed by the Scottish Executive to ensure logistics were in place to support the State Veterinary Service in dealing with infected premises and dangerous contacts and to support the armed services in dealing with the contiguous cull and pre-emptive sheep cull. He also promoted liaison between the armed services and state vets and took a key role in overseeing the 3km and contiguous cull in Dumfries and Galloway and the Birkshaw Forest mass disposal operation.

19. Dates and scale of military involvement

Operational in Dumfries and Galloway from 23 March 2001. Troops were deployed to Dumfries from the 52nd Lowland Brigade, 51st Highland Brigade and, from 29 March 2001, the 22nd Royal Artillery. They organised the transportation and destruction of carcasses for the 3km and contiguous culls. On 11 April 2001, the armed services set up a second operational base, at Newton Stewart, to deal with the outbreak in the Machars zone.

The number of soldiers deployed rose to a peak of around 470 in early April 2001.

Source: National Audit Office

The outbreak in Scotland continued

20. Pre-outbreak veterinary and related resources	Ayr Animal Health Division had 10 state vets, six animal health officers and 14 administrative and support staff. At the start of the outbreak, several state vets were sent on 'detached duty' to fight the disease in England.
	Galashiels had a complement of 8 state vets, 8 technical staff and 11.5 administrative staff.
21. Resources available at the height of the outbreak	In Dumfries and Galloway, peak staffing was in early May 2001. There were 180 vets, including 162 temporary veterinary inspectors, mainly drawn from Scottish private practices and agricultural colleges. There were also 62 animal health and field officers and 80 administrative and other support staff. Some 130 Dumfries and Galloway council staff supported the armed services and vets on a full-time basis.
	Galashiels had between 30-40 vets at the peak.
	Scotland was able to draw upon skilled Agricultural Officers from the Scottish Executive's Environment and Rural Affairs Department, who were accustomed to visiting farms, to work as field officers, for example serving Form D notices and supervising preliminary cleansing and disinfecting of affected farms. The Scottish Department's agricultural staff, as opposed to local authorities, carried out movement licensing.
22. Proportion of infected premises that tested positive for the disease	66%*.
	Based on results available for 169 infected premises.
23. Features of disease control	From 17 March 2001, there was pre-emptive slaughter of livestock traced from Longtown Market in Cumbria, including around 570 sheep in the Inverness area.
	From 22 March 2001 there was a cull of more than 400,000 sheep within 3 kilometres of infected premises.
	The contiguous cull, introduced on 26 March 2002, was applied to all contiguous premises at the leading edge of the advancing epidemic.
	Farmers' unions were generally supportive of the contiguous and 3km culls and standards of biosecurity by farmers were considered to be comparatively high.
	There were tight movement restrictions within the affected zone.
	There was early involvement of local authorities.
24. Proposals to vaccinate	In March and April 2001 vaccination was considered and contingency plans made but veterinary advice was that vaccination would not speed up eradication or prevent further incidence of disease and would take limited resources away from disease control operations. Vaccination did not have the support of the livestock industry and was not pursued.
25. Speed of slaughter on infected premises:	
• slaughtered-out within 24 hours of reported suspicions of disease	49% (Great Britain 41%).
• slaughtered-out in more than 24 but less than 36 hours	33% (Great Britain 32%).
• slaughtered-out in more than 36 but less than 48 hours	3% (Great Britain 6%).
• slaughtered-out in more than 48 hours	14% (Great Britain 22%).
	Based on data from 69 infected premises with full report and slaughter times available on the Disease Control System. The remaining premises did not have hours given for the reports of disease, but, from the dates given for report and slaughter, in only around 40% of these other cases was slaughter likely to have been achieved within 24 hours.

Source: National Audit Office

The outbreak in Scotland continued

26. Speed of slaughter on dangerous contact premises:	
• slaughtered-out within 48 hours of confirmation of related infected premises	14% (Great Britain 32%).
• slaughtered-out in more than 48 but less than 72 hours	13% (Great Britain 14%).
• slaughtered-out in more than 72 hours	73% (Great Britain 54%).
	Based on data from 862 dangerous contact premises with full report and slaughter times available on the Disease Control System.
27. Carcass disposal	Around 98% of carcasses from infected premises were disposed of by on-farm burns, the remaining 2%, comprising older cattle, were rendered in Motherwell. Around 1,400 sheep were buried on-farm, following a Scottish Environment Protection Agency site assessment. Greater on-farm burial was not possible because of thin soil and highly vulnerable aquifers (bodies of underground water) in the parts of Dumfries and Galloway affected by the outbreak. The Agency's policy was to consider carcass burial on a site-specific basis and to permit burial only where environmental conditions were acceptable and the relevant code of good agricultural practice could be met. The Agency advised against the use of certain materials on pyres, such as tyres, plastic materials or treated timber. The Fire Service advised on pyre construction.
	For the 3km and contiguous culls the Birkshaw Forest mass burial site was used extensively from 29 March 2001. More than 70% of non-infected premises carcasses were buried at Birkshaw. A further 6% were rendered and 22% burned. Before late April 2001, there were mass continuous burns at Hoddam quarry and East Riggs (on Ministry of Defence land), for Dumfries and Galloway, and Crook Knowes, near Jedburgh, for the Scottish Borders. Ash from the pyres has been buried in landfill sites and the impact on groundwater quality continues to be monitored.
	Four Scottish slaughterhouses were contracted for disposal for the Livestock Welfare (Disposal) Scheme.
28. Speed of disposal on infected premises:	
• disposed of within 24 hours of slaughter	29% (Great Britain 44%).
• in more than 24 but less than 48 hours	42% (Great Britain 13%).
• in more than 48 hours	29% (Great Britain 43%).
	Based on data from 142 infected premises with slaughter and disposal times available on the Disease Control System.
29. Speed of disposal on dangerous contact premises:	
• disposed of within 24 hours of slaughter	88% (Great Britain 71%).
• in more than 24 but less than 48 hours	9% (Great Britain 9%).
• in more than 48 hours	3% (Great Britain 20%).
	Based on data from 1,328 dangerous contact premises with slaughter and disposal times available on the Disease Control System.

Source: National Audit Office

The outbreak in Scotland continued

30. External communications:	On 2 March 2001, Scottish Executive and Dumfries and Galloway helplines were set up for FMD queries. Information was also provided on the Scottish Executive's website.
	Information letters were sent out by the Scottish Executive's Environment and Rural Affairs Department to livestock farmers. Regular stakeholder meetings were held in Edinburgh and Dumfries.
	The NFU Scotland also played an important role in disseminating information.
Costs 31. Cost to DEFRA	£334 million.
32. Average farm cleansing and disinfecting projected costs	£39,000 per farm in Dumfries and Galloway (Great Britain £35,600 per farm)[2].
33. Valuers' fees	In England and Wales, MAFF/DEFRA reached an agreement with the Central Association of Agricultural Valuers that valuers should be paid on the basis of 1% of stock value up to a maximum of £1,500 per day. However the Association did not represent valuers in Scotland where the Institute of Auctioneers and Appraisers in Scotland was the main representative body. DEFRA intended that the same arrangements for paying valuers should be in place in Scotland. However, the Ayr Disease Control Centre informed the Institute and firms of valuers that the fee to be paid would be based on 1% of the total valuation with a minimum fee of £500 per valuation and a maximum of £1,500 per valuation. Thus they were told that the minimum and maximum amounts would be on the basis of each valuation and not for each day. As a consequence there have been a number of disputes between DEFRA and valuers over payment. Valuers are claiming some £700,000 more than DEFRA believes they are entitled to.
34. Uncompensated costs estimated by DEFRA to:	
• Agricultural producers	£60 million.
• Food chain industries	£25 million.
35. Footpath closure and re-opening	Similar experiences to rest of Great Britain. Footpaths closed on 27 February 2001, following an Order made in the Scottish Parliament allowing local authorities and animal health inspectors to prevent access to footpaths and other land. From early March 2001 a risk assessment approach was adopted but there was genuine concern about the spread of the disease and footpaths only gradually reopened. On 23 March 2001 a model risk assessment was launched and a Comeback Code distributed. The Code was produced by Scottish Natural Heritage on behalf of the Executive. On 15 May 2001 guidance was sent to local authorities in Provisional Free Areas stipulating that footpaths could only be closed if supported by a risk assessment that satisfied the Department. On 24 May 2001, this access guidance was extended to all of Scotland except the Infected Area. By the end of June 2001, most local authorities had re-opened their rights of way.

Source: National Audit Office

Notes

[2] Cleansing and disinfecting costs are based on costs in October 2001. DEFRA is updating the figures.

18.6 Wales

The outbreak in Wales	
Context 1. Size and importance of the livestock sector	Pre-outbreak: 11.5 million sheep, 1.3 million cattle, and 0.1 million pigs. Agriculture contributed 1.4% of Wales' gross domestic product in 2000, with the livestock sector's share 59%. Exports accounted for 40% of Welsh lamb and sheep production.
Preparedness 2. Date local contingency plans last updated before the outbreak	Caernarfon Animal Health Divisional Office in July 2000; Cardiff in June 2000 and Carmarthen in August 2000.
3. Date of last simulation exercise	No recent test of the local contingency plan had been held, although one was being planned when the outbreak of classical swine fever occurred in East Anglia in late 2000, followed by FMD in February 2001. Because staff in Wales had been highly trained in preparation for impending disease control exercises, they were used in the classical swine fever outbreak in East Anglia. The remaining staff in Wales were rapidly overwhelmed when foot and mouth disease struck and consequently "the State Veterinary Service in Wales was not as prepared as it might have been to deal with an outbreak of foot and mouth disease" [National Assembly for Wales submission].
4. Involvement of stakeholders	Discussions had been held with local authorities on their role in an outbreak and they were to be involved in the exercise planned. Whilst their role had not been explored in detail in the local contingency plan it was expected that it would have become clearer if the exercises had taken place.
Course and extent of the outbreak 5. Date of confirmation of first case	27 February 2001 at the Welsh Country Foods abattoir in Gaerwen, Anglesey (identified on 25 February 2001 by an official veterinary surgeon). The first case on the mainland was confirmed on 28 February 2001 at Knighton, Powys.
6. Date of confirmation of last case	12 August 2001 at Crickhowell, Powys. The last case on Anglesey was confirmed on 24 March 2001.
7. Duration of outbreak between first and last cases	166 days. The outbreak in Wales was characterised by a succession of separate clusters of outbreaks with intervals between them.
8. Date declared free of the disease	4 December 2001. Anglesey was declared free of the disease in late August 2001.
9. Epidemiological groups and seeding	Four broad epidemiological groups: Anglesey (13 infected premises), north Powys (36 cases), south Powys (39 cases), and Welsh borders (including Monmouthshire and the Black Mountains) and South Wales Valleys (28 cases). In Anglesey, the disease was 'seeded' by infected animals brought from northern England to an abattoir. In the mainland, the disease was brought to Welshpool market by a contaminated vehicle that had been to Longtown market in Cumbria. Further south, another cluster was seeded by visits to a Herefordshire dealer who had been at Longtown market. There was subsequent spread through movements of farm personnel and vehicles.
10. Number of infected premises	117[1]
11. Number of dangerous contact premises slaughtered-out	713
12. Number of animals slaughtered on infected premises	70,000 – 87% sheep, 12% cattle and 1% pigs[1].

Source: National Audit Office

Notes

[1] Data on animals slaughtered and numbers of infected premises are based on DEFRA's information. There are some small differences compared with the figures that have been presented by National Assembly for Wales.

The outbreak in Wales continued

13. Number of animals slaughtered on dangerous contact and slaughter on suspicion premises	216,000 – 91% sheep, 8% cattle and 1% pigs. 51% of these animals were slaughtered on premises non-contiguous to infected premises and 42% on contiguous premises, and 7% were 'slaughter on suspicion' cases.
14. Number of animals slaughtered for welfare reasons	833,000, including 595,000 sheep, 199,000 'light lambs', 34,000 cattle and 5,000 pigs.
15. Proportion of country under Infected Area restrictions at one time	35%
Handling the outbreak 16. Animal Health arrangements	Under the Animal Health 1981 all functions for dealing with FMD rest with the Department since they were not devolved to the National Assembly for Wales in 1998. All employees of the State Veterinary Service in Wales report to the Department. Because of the legal requirement under the Animal Health Act 1981 for the Department and the National Assembly to implement legislation jointly in Wales, in practice the DEFRA took decisions affecting Wales in consultation with the devolved administration. The National Assembly's Rural Affairs Minister took an active role during the crisis in presenting policies decided in London and answering questions in the Assembly. On 26 March 2001, the National Assembly was asked by MAFF to establish an Operational Directorate on the lines of those set up in English Disease Control Centres, to support the State Veterinary Service. This was done under an agency agreement with MAFF, under Section 41 of the Government of Wales Act. All expenditure on FMD related issues came from DEFRA's vote.
17. Organisational structure during the 2001 outbreak	Disease Control Centres were set up at the Animal Health Divisional Offices in Caernarfon (for Anglesey) and Cardiff (for eastern and south-central Wales). The Llandrindod Wells area office served as an outreach control centre for cases in Powys. It reported to Cardiff, but from mid-April 2001 was given greater autonomy and was headed by a temporary Divisional Veterinary Manager. For serological testing in the Brecon Beacons, a temporary field centre was later set up. From 26 March 2001, a strategic Operations Centre was set up in the National Assembly's emergency operations room in Cathays Park, Cardiff. A Regional Operations Director drawn from the Assembly's staff headed the Centre. It co-ordinated the foot and mouth disease operation in Wales and was tasked with ensuring a multi-agency approach. The Operations Centre comprised 15 staff from the National Assembly for Wales, who operated under an agency agreement with the Department, and a similar number from the State Veterinary Service, military, police, the Environment Agency and, from 9 April, local authorities. The two main private sector contractors (Greyhound and MDW Transport) also had a liaison point at the Operations Centre.
18. Regional Operations Director: date of appointment and role	26 March 2001. The Regional Operations Director was a senior National Assembly official. He reported to the head of the Joint Co-ordinating Centre in the Department's headquarters, but operated under an understanding with the Department that he would consult and seek political guidance from Assembly Ministers.

Source: National Audit Office

19. Dates and scale of military involvement	Deployed from 26 March 2001. Soldiers from the 14 Signals Regiment were deployed in Anglesey, as well as Royal Air Force personnel. They became involved in unloading carcasses that it had been intended to burn on disused land adjacent to a RAF airfield at Mona. This plan was abandoned as a result of local opposition and successful negotiations on the availability of a suitable landfill site. On the mainland, troops came from 160 Brigade and the Household Cavalry and also included Gurkhas, who helped round up sheep in the Brecon Beacons. From mid-June 2001, the Household Cavalry were replaced by a small Territorial Army transport and logistics unit. At the height of the crisis more than 600 armed services personnel assisted, playing a key role in the logistics of slaughter and disposal, particularly for the contiguous cull.
20. Pre-outbreak veterinary and related resources	Cardiff Animal Health Division had eight full-time state veterinary officers: five at Cardiff and three at Llandrindod Wells. This was two below complement, but there were 2.5 temporary veterinary inspectors working on cattle tuberculosis cases. There were six animal health officers and 22 administrative staff. At the start of the outbreak, Cardiff Division lost three state vets on 'detached duty' to fight the disease in England, along with two animal health officers and some administrative staff. Caernarfon had four state vets (one below complement), along with the Divisional Veterinary Manager.
21. Resources available at the height of the outbreak	In Cardiff Division, there were 150 veterinary officers at the peak, chiefly temporary veterinary inspectors, recruited both locally and from overseas. Around 100 animal health officers and field staff, including staff from ADAS Consulting Ltd, and 200 administrative and other support staff were also involved. The latter included, in mid-April 2001, around 115 personnel provided by the National Assembly for Wales and administrative staff seconded from the Passport Agency. In Caernarfon there were up to 40 vets at the height of the local outbreak.
22. Proportion of infected premises that tested positive for the disease	59%* * Based on results available for 103 infected premises.
23. Features of disease control	In Anglesey there was a pre-emptive cull of 47,000 sheep in a 50 square mile area. On the mainland, the Chief Veterinary Officer made the decision that all sheep traded through Welshpool market on or after 19 February 2001 were to be culled. However in the light of a particular case, an infected premises at Llanfair Caereinion, where the tests came back negative, a decision was made to adjust the Welshpool cull to exclude lambs. There was intensive serological testing of sheep for understanding and control of the outbreak in the Brecon Beacons from June 2001, where risk of spread was increased by common grazing. A Movement Control Area was also introduced in the Brecon Beacons in July 2001 with local and long-distance movement licences revoked and intensified biosecurity monitoring. Bio-security standards among farmers were considered to be comparatively poor by DEFRA. This was partly a result of the structure and nature of livestock farming in some areas, with parcels of land held away from the home farm and movements of personnel to help out other farmers and for sheep shearing.

Source: National Audit Office

The outbreak in Wales continued

24. Proposals to vaccinate	In July and August 2001 the option of vaccinating all sheep in the Brecon Beacons National Park was discussed. The Cabinet Office Briefing Room advised against vaccination although agreed that Wales could adopt vaccination if the disease spread wider than anticipated. The vaccination option was not implemented as initial culling stamped out the disease.
25. Speed of slaughter on infected premises:	
• slaughtered-out within 24 hours of reported suspicions of disease	42% (Great Britain 41%).
• slaughtered-out in more than 24 but less than 36 hours	23% (Great Britain 32%).
• slaughtered-out in more than 36 but less than 48 hours	3% (Great Britain 6%).
• slaughtered-out in more than 48 hours	31% (Great Britain 22%).
	Based on data from 99 infected premises with full report and slaughter times available on the Disease Control System.
26. Speed of slaughter on dangerous contact premises:	
• slaughtered-out within 48 hours of confirmation of related infected premises	28% (Great Britain 32%).
• slaughtered-out in more than 48 but less than 72 hours	10% (Great Britain 14%).
• slaughtered-out in more than 72 hours	62% (Great Britain 54%).
	Based on data from 498 dangerous contact premises with full report and slaughter times available on the Disease Control System.
27. Carcass disposal	Around 62% of carcasses from infected premises were burned on-farm, 35% rendered and only 2% (chiefly sheep) were buried. The lack of clay and the reliance on private water supplies meant that on-farm burial was not normally an option. The National Assembly also stated that there should be no burial of cattle in Wales. Rendering was not used as much because of a lack of capacity and priority being given to Devon and Cumbria.
	Around a third of carcasses from non-infected premises were disposed of through burns, including mass burns at Eppynt, a further third by rendering and a quarter at landfill sites, including 43,000 sheep from the pre-emptive cull at the Penhesgyn landfill in Anglesey. A mobile air incinerator was used in the Welshpool area in May 2001. There were large public protests to the use of Eppynt, despite its remote location.
	Carcasses from the Livestock Welfare (Disposal) Scheme were disposed of mainly in landfill sites.
28. Speed of disposal on infected premises:	
• disposed of within 24 hours of slaughter	62% (Great Britain 44%).
• in more than 24 but less than 48 hours	12% (Great Britain 13%).
• in more than 48 hours	26% (Great Britain 43%).
	Based on data from 108 infected premises with slaughter and disposal times available on the Disease Control System.

Source: National Audit Office

The outbreak in Wales continued

29. Speed of disposal on dangerous contact premises:	
• disposed of within 24 hours of slaughter	78% (Great Britain 71%).
• in more than 24 but less than 48 hours	8% (Great Britain 9%).
• in more than 48 hours	14% (Great Britain 20%). *Based on data from 710 dangerous contact premises with slaughter and disposal times available on the Disease Control System.*
30. External communications	The National Assembly set up helplines on 27 February 2001. Helplines were also set up later in Divisional Offices. Over 100,000 calls were taken by the helplines in Wales during the crisis. A communications strategy unique to Wales was implemented. This established 44 local public information points across Wales and a programme of mailshots to farmers on a variety of foot and mouth disease related issues (51 factsheets and 16 advisory letters were sent). Information was also provided on the Assembly's website. In Cardiff, from early on, Assembly Ministers gave regular briefing sessions with stakeholders and there were regular meetings with local authorities, farmers and farmers' unions. Senior officials also had many meetings with farmers to explain what was happening. In Caernarfon, there were daily liaison meetings with enforcement authorities and farmers' unions.
Costs 31. Cost to DEFRA	£102 million.
32. Average farm cleansing and disinfecting projected costs	£44,000 per farm (Great Britain £35,600 per farm)[2].
33. Valuers' fees	Similar arrangements to England. DEFRA took the lead in dealing with this issue because of their legal functions under the Animal Health Act 1981.
34. Uncompensated costs estimated by DEFRA to:	
• Agricultural producers	£65 million.
• Food chain industries	£25 million.
35. Footpath closure and re-opening	On 27 February 2001 an Order was made enabling local authorities to make blanket closures of footpaths. On 20 March 2001 the National Assembly for Wales issued guidance to local authorities and the public on what activities could be undertaken in the countryside without adding to the risks of spreading the disease. Guidance issued on 23 May 2001 encouraged local authorities to re-open all public footpaths, except those near infected premises. By the end of June 2001 most local authorities had re-opened their rights of way.

Source: National Audit Office

Notes

[2] Cleansing and disinfecting costs are based on costs in October 2001. DEFRA is updating the figures and the cost for Wales is expected to fall to around £38,000.

18.7 The Inquiry Secretariat

Seconded from:

Alun Evans,
Secretary to the Inquiry   Department for Transport

Nicola Baker	Department for Trade and Industry
Rupert Cazalet	Legal Secretariat to the Law Officers
Dominic Fagan	Cabinet Office
Lucy Harington	Contract staff
Matthew Hill	Cabinet Office
Jane Mardell	Department for Education and Skills
Siân Simpkins	Cabinet Office
Dr Min-Min Teh	Unilever PLC
Patrick Wall	Contract staff
Sue Wilson	Department for Transport

We would like to thank the Policy Commission and Royal Society for their co-operation throughout our Inquiry. In addition, we would like to thank the National Audit Office for giving us permission to reproduce material from their report, and the staff of other departments for their assistance, particularly the Inquiry Liaison Unit at DEFRA.

We would like to thank The Mirror for permission to reproduce its front page of 26 April 2001.

We would also like to thank the following for their expert advice:

Professor John Kay
Dr John Ryan
Professor Bernard Silverman
Professor Michael Winter

And Peter Whitehurst for his legal advice to the Inquiry.

Inquiry visits

The Inquiry made the following regional visits:

22-24 January 2002	South West
5-7 February 2002	Wales
13-15 February 2002	Scotland
4-6 March 2002	North East
11-13 March 2002	Cumbria and the North West
3-5 April 2002	Yorkshire

The Inquiry also made visits to The Netherlands, France and the European Commission in Brussels.

Printed in the UK by The Stationery Office Limited
On behalf of the Controller of Her Majesty's Stationery Office
ID 97807   759856   7/02   19585